I Woke Up One Day
And Changed My F★cking Mind

I WOKE UP ONE DAY AND CHANGED MY F*CKING MIND

By Challaine

Copyright © 2024 Challaine
Paperback Edition

All rights reserved. No part of this publication may be reproduced, distributed, or transmitted in any form or by any means, including photocopying, recording, or other electronic or mechanical methods, without the prior written permission of the publisher, except in the case of brief quotations embodied in critical reviews and certain other noncommercial uses permitted by copyright law.

Table of Contents

Introduction		vii
CHAPTER 1	'90s Girl	1
CHAPTER 2	Remember When	7
CHAPTER 3	Who Am I Without Jungle Juice?	21
CHAPTER 4	Why Do I Keep Poisoning Myself?	35
CHAPTER 5	Fucking Childhood Trauma	49
CHAPTER 6	My First Drink	59
CHAPTER 7	The Pain	67
CHAPTER 8	What Do I Do Now?	75
CHAPTER 9	Rock Bottom	77
CHAPTER 10	Consumption At Its Finest	83
CHAPTER 11	Social Celebrities	89
CHAPTER 12	Sobriety… What Does It Actually Mean?	93
CHAPTER 13	Christmas House	97
CHAPTER 14	An Evolution	101
CHAPTER 15	Authentically Free	107
CHAPTER 16	The How, Who, What, Where, but MOST importantly HOW?	125
CHAPTER 17	Quitting Cold Turkey VS Drinking Responsibly	143
CHAPTER 18	Accountability	155
CHAPTER 19	Lessons Learned	173

CHAPTER 20	Keep Growing and Going	189
CHAPTER 21	Evolution Of Personal Growth	197
CHAPTER 22	Mindful Path To Recovery	217
CHAPTER 23	Self-Reflection	233
CHAPTER 24	Overcoming Obstacles	241
CHAPTER 25	Have The Best Day Ever!	247
A Letter To My Beautiful Children		251
Acknowledgements		263

Introduction

*I Woke Up One Day & Changed My F*cking Mind* is a compelling and introspective; imperfectly perfect story that chronicles my transformative journey through sobriety that "only" took 20 years. As I'm always reminded, "You will continue to be taught the same lessons until they are learned." I'm not sure why it took me so long, especially after many, what people would call "rock bottoms," such as my arrest. My lesson was finally learned on January 16, 2024.

I'm about to take you on a real-time journey of quitting alcohol, reliving my past, healing emotionally and physically, while looking toward what lies ahead. You will be getting sober with me in a sense.

My story unfolds as a personal mind purge, providing a raw and authentic account of the challenges, triumphs, and profound insights gained while breaking free from the grips of alcohol.

It is my hope that I am able to connect with others who have been on a similar journey to mine as "functioning alcoholics", and to those in recovery still utilizing as many resources as possible to help them stay on the path to health and living free. I even hope to reach those who are still heavily into the bottle and somehow came across this book and it now sits in your bathroom and is your "shit reading." Whatever the case may be, whatever is going on in your head about your relationship with alcohol, believe it or not, we need a community. Whether it is a silent community i.e., reading others' stories on their journey through alcohol use and abuse, perusing Facebook and watching sobriety reels. Or maybe you are looking for an active community of AA, therapy or talking with friends and family.

My goal is to be a part of your community in some sort of way. I want to give you inspiration, hope, love, compassion and guidance (only based on my own personal journey). Please note that I am NOT a medical practitioner, nor am I a licensed Therapist. Although I am an experienced ex-alcoholic of 20+ years and have my own personal journey and guidance to share with the world, now that I am finally sober.

I'm here to share my journey, my recovery and self-discovery while being of service to others. It's worth a mention that there are topics that can be triggering to some. I'm not going to censor them but I do talk about my own personal molestation, getting arrested, heavy substance abuse as well as talk of death and suicide. I felt super uncomfortable reliving some of my memories, but there's no pussy footin' around here. I'm either doing this or I'm not.

It's tough to talk about having a problem with alcohol especially when I appeared so put together to the outside world. Inside, I was in shambles – mentally and physically. I had (and sometimes still do) a pretty hard shell of an exterior but inside I was an absolute disaster. Does any of this sound familiar? Good! Then you have come to the right place. I am your community.

This book encapsulates my candid observations with my relationship with alcohol, diving into the pivotal moments that led to the decision to embrace a life of sobriety. It wasn't just one in particular but a culmination of a lifetime of shitty events.

As I navigate the complexities of withdrawal and the emotional fuckery of recovery, I hope you find yourself within these pages and have true solace in knowing that I am here with you, I feel you and understand you. You are here to witness the gradual emergence of self-discovery and resilience as I become sober.

Throughout this book, I reflect on the multifaceted impacts of sobriety on various aspects of my life and how the fuck I'm getting through them. I'm sharing my experiences with you as a

Introduction

"90s Girl" and what it was like growing up in that time. Talking about my past childhood traumas from an emotionally disconnected mother, to being molested and her not believing me as she states I was "acting out for attention." I share our statements (hers and mine) from the police report from when I was 13 of the "alleged incident", as she puts it.

I dive into the connections that were surrounded by alcohol and a party lifestyle, and mending relationships such as those with my kids and partner. I rediscovered personal passions (like journaling, which then turned into this book), all the while pursuing a more holistic and soul connected self. With that said – no, I'm not going to preach to you to find Jesus and start hugging trees. Although by all means if that helps you in your recovery then I fully support you and hold zero judgement. Just like our journeys through alcoholism are completely different, so will our journeys of recovery. As long as you get to the end of your journey going through the process and coming out better than you once were, you have made it. Don't we all want to just make it?

I Woke Up One Day & Changed My F*cking Mind doesn't shy away from addressing the societal stigmas associated with addiction, offering a poignant observation of how the fuck did so many of us get to this point? Nevermind Covid19, there's a bigger pandemic happening silently in the background. There are so many of us who just want to be free. I'm here to let you know. If I can do it after 20 years, you can do it too. If you haven't yet it's just cuz you aren't truly ready and/or haven't found the right tools externally or internally to help you along the way.

I share insights into the role of support systems, both personally and professionally. Fostering a sense of accountability and providing strength during moments of vulnerability.

We get into the practical aspects of maintaining sobriety, offering guidance on setting boundaries, cultivating healthy coping mechanisms, and navigating social situations without relying on substances. Throughout this very personal labour of love, I emphasise the importance of mindfulness, self-reflection, and continuous personal growth in the ongoing journey of recovery with a few (well many) f bombs along the way.

As my story unfolds, you will witness my setbacks, milestones, other addictions and celebrations (I hope). Each is a testament to the resilience and determination required to embrace a life without alcohol. It's fucking hard but it's definitely possible.

There's lots of juicy content in between these pages but this book concludes with a hopeful vision of the future – a future rich in authentic connections, personal fulfilment, and a deep appreciation for the clarity that sobriety brings. Definitely for me, but I'm hopeful it's for you too…

*I Woke Up One Day & Changed My F*cking Mind* is not just a personal memoir but a guide and source of inspiration for those contemplating or undergoing their own journey to sobriety. Through my honesty, vulnerability and education, this book serves as an important tool to add to your arsenal. This is for anyone seeking a life of meaning and free from the constraints of alcohol.

Even though I hope this book reaches so many people, I was initially intrigued to reach out and connect with moms (as I'm a mother of four), my peers who I "know" and who "know" me such as my fellow '90s girls, my sisters from other misters.

Although after lots of thought and reflection, I opened my mind and want to write these words to not only those who can relate and are sick of the fucking roller coaster of drinking but also to a younger generation. In a sense, to my younger self.

Looking back (hindsight is always 20/20, isn't it?) There weren't many resources for teens/young adults that were captivating, raw and that really showed what the effects of alcohol can have on you in your present and future. All I remember were the MADD Canada ads on TV (Mothers Against Drunk Driving). While these campaigns were definitely helpful in becoming aware of the risks of such behaviour, no one ever talked about the mental and physical effects from alcohol such as depression and anxiety for the long term. Not once was I ever told if I kept drinking that I would want to end my life! I'm sorry but this is a BIG deal! Well, now it's time. Let's fucking talk about it and all of the other nasty shit that comes with prolonged alcohol use.

I aim to have this book edited as little as possible. As I mentioned I got sober while writing this book in January of 2024. I was originally going to title it *'90s Girl-My Journey Through Alcoholism, Sobriety and Living Authentically Free*. I have been witness to so many women my age, my peers battling this fucking demon. So we start there.

Although as I recover, grow and expand my consciousness to my new sober reality I don't want to put generational limitations on myself as to who I can connect with or who can connect with me. I'm 38 at the time of writing this book. If some 50-year-old broad is a potty mouth like me and picked up my book cuz it said fuck on the front, then we have something in common.

Alright, Challaine, deep breath in ….
Deep breath out.
There's literally no going back now.
I love you, you got this!

CHAPTER 1
'90s Girl

Hey, '90s Girl – Yep, you! I see you. You stick out in a crowd like a sore thumb. That's okay – I do too. It's a whole thing.

Let's have a chat. We're gettin' old, eh? We're like allllmost 40 or allllllmost close to 50. Men in in their 50's and early 60's are fuckin' sexy! Can anyone say John Stamos? At the time of this writing he is 60! That's absolutely nuts.

Many of us have 1-6 kids now, and are metaphorically counting down the time on our "clock." "I want more kids, I don't want more kids." The mental battle back and forth of "I'm getting too old, I've got teenagers now, starting over? Absolutely Not."

"But, babies!!! They are just the most breathtaking little beings on this planet. Okay! I'm going to do it. But then… What about my career? More daycare? My kids can stay home by themselves now."

What about breaking your "oldish" body to do it again? For me it's my hips – my fucking hips. There's no way they could support another one. But… babies!

What about knowing you can't have your wine every night when you cook supper because drinking when you are pregnant is just plain stupid?

Have you switched careers, about 6-10 times like me? I went from Paramedic School (I graduated but didn't take the final practical exam because I was chicken shit), to Photography, to Personal Training, Holistic Practitioner, Natural Nutritionist, to MULTIPLE mlm's, to launching my own fitness clothing line, to owning two Home Service based businesses. I'm also currently registered and have completed 3 out of 12 (I think) modules for Interior Design. I have registered but not completed a Landscaping course, Registered and on module one for Real Estate and NOW writing my damn book. Shiny object syndrome anyone? With all of that, after years and years, I've finally connected to my soul and am fulfilling my own dharma.

I bet some of your friends' parents have died, or maybe even your parents have passed away? Are you also coming across on social media some peers from high school who have passed on? It's such a bizarre time we are in.

Doesn't high school feel like a lifetime ago in your day-to-day reality but it's also just right around the corner, not a long distant memory? Does part of you still feel like you are there – walking down those halls with your whole future ahead of you, and that things haven't changed? That you will all see each other again?

It's weird but the reality is that it's over. Those thoughts are challenging, it's sad, some of it is happy. I went to three junior highs in the same year and then one high school. No wonder I never felt like I "fit in" going to three schools in three years at the age of 12/13. The most awkward years in a young teenage girl's life.

Does this past and present leave you stuck in this mind and body that you don't know or recognize? Like your body is getting older but you are still that young, fun, partying, invincible teenager or young 20 something? That being in this state of push and pull has you absolutely exhausted? You are just trying to figure your shit out, make some money, raise a few babies (or not) and just be happy? Don't you just want to be happy? I get it! So do I (spoiler alert – I am. Now).

Does any of this sound kinda familiar?

You are maybe in a blended family. Once? Twice? I like to say that a blended family is the new modern day family. I'm in my second blended family and I wouldn't change it for anything. This is after asking the father of my first two to leave. Our relationship lasted seven years. But then we stopped thriving as a couple. We had turned into roommates and our friendship crumbled. It broke both of us. He was my best friend, and father to my babies! I loved him so much but the passion was gone and I wasn't IN love with him anymore.

Then I was with such a wonderful and amazing man who helped shape and raise my first two for five years. He came into my life when my oldest was three and my youngest at the time was six months old. We were together for five years and had one of the most amazing relationships I could have ever asked for. He was not only my superman but superman in his community. He was loved so hard because he was so selfless and loved hard in return. Our time came to an end in May 2017, and then he took his own life in 2022. On my dad's birthday. Rest in peace, Will. "Until I see you again."

As mentioned, I'm in my second blended family relationship which I get into more detail as we move through these pages.

Okay, back to being oldish. Is it starting to hurt yet when you get out of bed? Do you loathe going out to the club now, cuz guess what? You're not the hot chick in the bar anymore! If you have to put on your eye cream before your make up – you have officially moved into the cougar phase of your life.

You're now the mom with the Bailey's in her mug at the hockey rink at 7am. I know you mom, I am she. Gotta keep warm!

I know my son is going to read this at some point in his life, or at least hear about it. The Bailey's was on occasion. I want him to know that I wasn't drinking every time I was at the rink at 7am, but it definitely did happen a couple of times.

Has your life blown up in your face more than once? Of course it has, but you made it through and you're here to talk about it. Oh and also because you're a '90s girl and a fucking badass who conquers every single demon that shows up in your life. Sometimes with grace, sometimes not but always with fortitude!

So, why me and why this book?

Because sometimes it's nice to know that someone else has gone through or is going through something similar to you. It's nice to not have to talk to your therapist, or your friends and family, but just a stranger that will listen.

Have you ever been out (usually drinking) at a club called something like "The Back Alley" or "Cowboys" and you share your whole life story with someone while out for a smoke? You probably shared too much, jumped up and down and said, "Oh, my God, me too" and so did they. You two were probably around the same age. You may have cried a little, and so did they. You girls hugged it out, fixed each other's mascara in one hand while holding your heels from "Shoe Dazzle" in the other and then it was time for you to take off with the guy you met that night. Or perhaps your girlfriends threw you in a taxi and gave the driver your address, cuz you were too wasted and needed to put yourself to bed. But you weren't too wasted to eat that slice of pizza with ranch sauce from the little hole in the wall pizza shop that stayed open until 4am. Let's be honest. It was usually puked up by the next morning

Wasn't it nice to just pour all those feelings out to a complete stranger? Well, that's what I'm doing here – knowing full well that the majority of my readers are strangers, and I'm going to feel fucking awesome about it. I'm going to share like the drunk girl at the bar. I'm going to tell you some secrets, my fuck ups, my wins, my losses and all the messy bits in between. But as I do this I've got slippers on, not high heels.

This book is about my journey through alcoholism starting at a young age, sobriety and living authentically free. Part of it is about growing up in the '90s and what it's like living as a '90s girl in 2024.

This is a memoir of sorts, a collection of moments and memories that have shaped who I am today. It's not going to be pretty, but it's going to be real. And I hope that by sharing my story, it can help someone else who may be going through something similar. I mean that's the ultimate goal. I have always been one to help where I can. I hope this book reaches the right eyes to help the soul.

I hope that you find this to be a book that you can connect with, as I know my journey is personal but it's also relatable. My narrative provides a raw and authentic account of the challenges, triumphs, and profound insights gained while breaking free from the grip of alcohol, formerly known as jungle juice (that's what I used to tell my kids it was called when they were little). Ridiculous. It was a crazy juice that only Mummy could have.

The book begins with a candid exploration of my stupid relationship with alcohol, getting into the pivotal moments that led to the decision to embrace a life of sobriety. A lot of what I will share comes from a place of deep reflection as I write, a lot of what I like to call *"Brain Wow"* moments. You can maybe relate to a *Brain Wow* as Oprah coined the term an *"Aha Moment."*

As I navigate the complexities of withdrawal and the emotional turbulence of recovery, you my fellow boozers, will witness the gradual emergence of self-discovery and resilience. This is what I aspire for you to take in for yourself: acceptance, growth, forgiveness and a bright fulfilling future.

I have included many lists and the impacts of sobriety on various aspects of life. From forging authentic connections and mending relationships to rediscovering personal passions and pursuing a holistic well-being.

This book doesn't shy away from addressing the societal stigmas associated with addiction, offering a poignant view through empathy and understanding. It's always been such a social norm to see booze all around us. It's been ingrained in us since such an early age that it was appropriate to drink as an adult. That a glass of wine (for me it was a bottle + per night) or a six-pack of beer was the norm to have after work every day. I will share with you some insights into the role of support systems, both personal and professional, in fostering a sense of accountability and providing strength during moments of vulnerability and how we don't have to fit the societal mold anymore.

We get into the practical aspects of maintaining sobriety, offering guidance on setting boundaries, cultivating healthy coping mechanisms, and navigating social situations without relying on substances. Throughout, I will emphasize the importance of mindfulness, self-reflection, and continuous personal growth in the ongoing journey of recovery.

As my story unfolds, you, my sisters from another mister, will witness some milestones and celebrations. Each is a testament to the resilience and determination required to embrace a life without alcohol. My goal is to conclude with a hopeful vision of the future – a future rich in authentic connections, personal fulfilment, and a deep appreciation for the clarity that sobriety brings for you, my beautiful reader, and me.

This is not just another book about being sober, nor is it just a personal memoir but a guide and source of inspiration for those contemplating or undergoing their own journey through sobriety. I've put my heart on my sleeve to share with the world.

This is for you my fellow '90s girl, still figuring life out and taking the journey one day at a time. I feel you. I see you.

I am you!

CHAPTER 2
Remember When

Sorry, I forgot to introduce myself. "How Rude."

I'm Challaine. An almost 40-year-old Canadian mum of four ridiculously amazing kids. They are 15, 12, 2 and 1. Two boys and two girls. I must have been an angel in my past life to be so blessed now to call them mine. Good Lord, almost 40. That seems so crazy. My life is moving so fast…

I'm pretty low key. I love my sweats, tank tops, big comfy sweaters, wine, cooking, scrapbooking, gardening, wine, cleaning, organizing, wine, grocery shopping and wine.

I like to keep my circle small. I've had some of the greatest best friends over the years, though. They have been so incredibly loyal and faithful to me. I need to give a shout out to my best friends who have supported me over the past 20 years. I wouldn't be who I am today without them: Canadian Club Whiskey and ginger ale, Twisted Tea, Captain Morgan, Caesar (like a Bloody Mary), Michelada, Vodka Cran and Vodka Water. We can't forget about my favourite bestie – Wine!

I welcomed them all into my life but as with any relationship that becomes toxic we had to call it quits. The therapy didn't work to keep us together. It took a while but I finally grew the cojones to initiate the break up. They are pissed though. They keep knocking at my door, trying to apologize, trying to say they have changed, trying to negotiate, committing to cleaning up their mess if they can come back. They have always been so trusting in me. I should return the favour, shouldn't I? I mean it's always an option.

Now you obviously picked up this book for a reason. Something has resonated within you just by looking at the title. So I guess I made it catchy enough. Good.

What has come up for you so far? Does it feel weird? Did you relive some moments? Can you remember those times? Painful? Funny? Stay with me, I've got a ton of '90s memories coming right up.

Are you a '90s girl, or are pretty close to it? We're a rare breed. It's not like we are a huge global society. What years are considered to be a '90s child? If you were born in 1985-1994 (basically "growing up" in the '90s) you are considered to be a "90s child." Here's some fun stats on what a rare breed we are. In Canada there were only 1,599,653 baby girls born within these years (www150.statcan.gc.ca).

You are LITERALLY 1 in an almost one million, my fellow Canadian Girls.

To my girls in the states and around the world, don't worry, you are rare too, lol. To pull up all those stats, is for another book. I do, however, encourage you to look it up on your country's statistics website. It's quite interesting. I'm curious to see what you come up with!

The world is a different place than when we grew up. Social media didn't exist. I mean we had MSN messenger on ALL THE TIME. Do you remember getting off the bus and rushing home to go straight to your computer and sign in to talk to all the people you were just in school with? Omg, lol.

Remember when we had to ask permission from our parents before using the house phone? What about picking up another phone when they were on it talking to their friends. I got in shit one day from my mum's friend. She KNEW I was on the line listening in and I remember her screaming at me and threatening me that she was coming right over to smack me! Moms in the '90s had no filters and they were absolute badasses.

She never actually did smack me but the threat was enough for me to quietly hang up the phone.

2. Remember When

Remember when we had to make plans and actually stick to them because there were no cell phones to text saying "I'll be late"? We had to rely on our friends to take actual pictures of us on a camera, get them developed at the store and then put them in an album or scrapbook (remember those)? It was me. I was that person. I still have every single picture that I ever took. Some people like to burn their memories. I've got a ton of shitty ones but they are a part of what has shaped me.

Life just felt simpler back then. But maybe that's just the nostalgia talking. Is life really harder now with so many conveniences? Are we just illusioned by the past because we were younger and didn't have mortgages, car payments, kids? We did have bullies, family drama, poverty, sick parents, emotionally detached parents, only child syndrome, pressure in school (I did anyways). As I type this out, I'm not sure that "back then" was easier. It was still hard, just in a different way. It's a matter of subjectivity, I suppose.

I grew up in Calgary Alberta, home of the world famous Calgary Stampede. I think it's something like a million people from all around the world come to my city and get wasted for 10 days. It's a pretty big deal with concerts and cowboys.

When we were little we didn't have a ton of options for things to do – but that was okay. We made our own fun. We rode bikes, played outside until the sun went down, drank out of the hose and got lost in our imaginations. We didn't need technology to keep ourselves entertained.

But with that simplicity there was also curiosity. Curiosity about alcohol, the "unknown." I put that in quotations because we knew about it through our parents, and would have a sip here and there but it tasted awful. There must have been something to it though as our parents were drinking it all the time. Homemade wine, anyone?

As early as junior high school, alcohol was a constant presence at parties and gatherings. Lots of bush parties, a random house party here and there. Let's be honest, not many kids in junior high get the whole house to themselves for a weekend very often.

It was a normal thing to drink and get drunk on a Saturday night, only to regret it on Sunday morning. And so the cycle began. Couldn't wait for the weekend!

I loved to dance. I loved boys – a few in particular. I loved to drink and I loved to have a good time.

Being a '90s girl (in hindsight) was fucking awesome! But it also fucking sucked! When I think of my childhood, it's not all too thrilling. It kind of stings to go back there.

Or did you have an absolutely incredible childhood? Sorry, I don't talk about that too much as I'm unable to relate. Most of my past is super uncomfortable to relive. It just gives me this icky and awkward feeling. If your childhood was amazing that makes me so happy for you! I wish it was the same for me, although my past is my past and if I didn't have it then I wouldn't be who I am today: a happy, confident and sober woman.

REMEMBER WHEN

I've compiled a list of "remember whens." I hope this takes your mind away for a few minutes and puts a smile on your face. This list is one I talk about often with my best friend Tori. Here we go…

Let's go on a little trip together. No, no, not that kind of trip – that comes later. I meant a trip down memory lane.

My pretty little line up of Remember Whens…

Do you remember having a pager cuz your parents couldn't afford a cell phone? Hell, they could hardly afford to call across the nation before 6pm.

Subtitles – Remember when your parents would watch TV with the subtitles on? I bet you do it now! I know I certainly do. If I can't read the TV, I can't hear it.

Remember lying on the floor, or your bed with your legs up on the wall talking for HOURS with your best friend?

2. Remember When

Remember the see through phone where you could see all the cool colourful wires inside? Or maybe you had one of the matte V Tech phones. My best friend had the cool one, I had the V Tech. This was later when we were FINALLY allowed phones in our rooms.

Before that, remember the main land line being attached to a 20-foot cord that you wedged in the door of your room so you could talk privately about boys, your teacher that you had a weird giddy crush on or the cool girls who were such bitches?

Remember rushing home to check the caller ID and answering machine just in case a boy called and left a message? DELETE! Of course you had juuuust enough time to do this before Full House came on at four o'clock.

Hellooooo, Uncle Jesse! Twenty years later, and he's still my all time celebrity crush. But now with that salt and pepper hair and a few wrinkles. "Owww, owww, have mercy!"

P.S. My husband's celebrity crush is Sofia Vergara – Fair... She's a babe!

Remember staying out until the street lights came on?

Remember tobogganing for hours until you were absolutely frozen and came in for hot chocolate? The burning in your fingers as they warmed up? I remember lying on the heat register to thaw.

Remember singing your heart out to Mariah Carey's "Hero" or "Always Be My Baby?" What about Celine Dion's "All By Myself" or "My Heart Will Go On?" Remember singing those songs on full blast and hitting every single note (not actually, though)?

Remember being sooo good that you were going to be a singer when you grew up? Tori & I were so good that we made demo tapes. Our band name was "Silver." We also started a dance group called the Peace Keepers. Omg, lol.

Remember going door to door on Halloween with the Unicef boxes around your neck that would get loaded with pennies?

Remember jumping all the ropes for all the hearts? Yes, I admit, I did pocket a bit of that money. I thought I deserved a bit of cash to go to the 7-11 (Sev as we called it and still do) after all of that door knocking. Plus we literally didn't have jobs but had shit to buy. Five cent candies were my jam! I can't believe they have doubled in price since I was young. What a gyp!

Did you ever steal from a store? I did! It was usually makeup. I remember stealing a bunch of makeup with Tori from a grocery store called Co-Op and we made it through the parking lot – to the bus stop and thought we were safe, until we weren't and were taken back by security. I have a lifetime ban from that store. I wonder if they would remember me if I walk in?

Remember the wooden and metal playgrounds? It was either splinters or burns. There's this meme going around on the socials about playgrounds, with a merry go round, a teeter totter, a slide and monkey bars. It basically asks which one did you get hurt on? For me it was the monkey bars (trying to jump to the 4th bar and falling onto my back and getting winded). I can still feel the terror from that moment.

Remember getting into fights with your best friend and it crushed your world to see them hanging out with someone else? There was no social media back then so there was no way to creep on them. I can feel this moment in my gut.

Remember when one of you had to awkwardly call the other one (on the landline) for "something" that your mom needed (not really) – but that broke the ice and you were best friends again?

Remember going through the Delia's magazine listening to one of your penny CDs from Columbia House, and wanting every single outfit? Oh! The outfits. It's funny how it's come full circle! The platforms, crop tops and wide leg jeans are back. I'm reliving my young fashion through my 12-year-old daughter. It's interesting how the apple doesn't fall far from the tree.

2. Remember When

Remember the party lines that you had to be eighteen to call into? I wonder what would have happened if I didn't actually meet the guy I was chatting with on the party line. I ended up having my first drink with him then eventually my mother moved us to another province to get me away from him. I loved him hard and it absolutely crushed me to leave him and my Tori.

Remember doing your makeup and getting so dressed up to go to the mall to check out boys and stay for HOURS just window shopping or only having like $60 to spend but somehow ended up with a stash of really rad things? A stolen T-shirt or two may have made it into the bags. Our favourite stores were Music World, HMV, Mariposa, Bootlegger and Le Chateau. I can't stand the mall now. Times sure have changed.

Remember bumpin' around town on public transit with your Walkman (or Discman) and headphones? Tori and I used to ride the transit for hours!

Remember swimming with your best friend at the leisure centre until you wanted to puke? We (yes, Tori) would spend like eight hours at the wave pool – stop halfway through for some poolside fries then get right back in. Again, to watch all the boys!

Remember your first concert being the Backstreet Boys and just BALLING when you saw them live? Nick Carter was always my favourite. I was about 11 when I went to my first BSB concert with Tori. The hype was absolute pandemonium. Standing in the freezing cold since 6 am. We were so bored, so fucking cold! Her dad ended up bringing us mitts and scarves, which we ended up just pitching in the venue when the show started.

Remember line dancing to "Cadillac Ranch" in elementary school? Maybe it's an Alberta thing, or even a Canadian thing but why did they make us do that in gym class? Okay, in all fairness it totally paid off when I was in my early 20s and attending all of the country music concerts and bars. You could count on me to lead the line dance at Cowboys.

Remember the school assemblies with all of the classrooms lining up in the hallway and making their way to the gymnasium? "Shhhh, quiet." I can still hear the teachers with their fingers to their lips. We would all mosey into the gym to sit on the floor for an hour. I swear the teachers probably hated assembly time. It probably took more work to get us ducks all in a row than it took for the actual assembly.

Remember when they didn't lock all of the school doors? According to lockoutusa.com there's now three levels of lockdowns. What the actual f?

A Level 1 lockdown means that there is a threat (shooter, criminal, etc.) nearby, but not necessarily targeting the school itself. The school will be locked until law enforcement officials state that everything is clear.

A Level 2 lockdown means that the threat is on the property and more likely to cause harm. Students and educators should immediately barricade themselves in the nearest room and stay quiet.

A Level 3 lockdown refers to life-threatening danger. In other words, there is a threat on the property that is seeking to cause harm immediately. Even in this situation, everyone should remain calm and wait for the police to signal.

That literally blows my mind. We didn't have anything like this growing up! When my kids talk about their lockdown procedures at school it's still so foreign to me. I am grateful though that they have their cellphones and can contact me when this shit happens. My daughter has called me before in regards to a serious danger on the school grounds and they were locked in. Needless to say, I did pick her up that day and kept her home the next.

Remember when your friend had a birthday party and you listened to and danced around in your Spice Girls outfits and you would fight over who got to be which Spice? Do you still have your Aqua and Hanson CDs in a binder with the rest of your burnt CDs? I certainly do.

2. Remember When

Do you remember getting bullied for being too fat, having a pig nose, chubby hands, bucked teeth, awkwardly bleached hair? Did you get bullied for where you lived? What about wearing second hand or handmade clothes? Were you embarrassed by the family vehicle? No? Just me? I was bullied hard in elementary school for my pig nose and fat hands. It's still ingrained in me now, which is terrible I know, although I definitely don't hide my hands up in my sleeves anymore.

Did you end up switching schools in junior high because you got bullied so hard? I was in three junior high schools. I was bullied in two of them, skipped one then bullied again by a bunch of NEW assholes in high school. Kids are so fucking mean. After my first Junior High switch (that same year) my mother moved us away to another province. She took me from my Tori. It was just like the movies, bawling as I looked in the rearview mirror. I was so pissed at my mother.

Remember the first time you smoked pot and drank bootlegged "Lucky" beer or 2L coolers out in the boonies? Where did we tell our parents we were going, and how did none of them realize we were absolutely wasted when we got home? Maybe they did know, but were silently teaching us a lesson by not smacking us upside the head, knowing that the hangover we would be feeling would be punishment enough.

It's interesting the little tidbits of history that stick with you, and these events are the ones that we rely on which determine who we are and how they have shaped us. What about all of the other events in our lives that were so prevalent at the time but now we can't even dig deep enough to find them? Where do they go? The memories may be gone but the events were real and must have contributed to who we are today.

Above were a few of my '90s memories. It's uncomfortably comfortable to relive some of those. But relive I did and I'll continue to do so as I move forward in this book. All in the name of writing my story. That's the thing about being authentically free. It requires vulnerability. It requires cracking yourself open and exposing the ugly, hurtful and real parts of you. There's definitely a lot of that throughout these pages.

But it also means embracing the good, the funny, and the happy moments too. So as we go on this journey together, let's remember to hold space for both the darkness and the light. I'll hold it for you, if you hold it for me. Hey! Like I always say, "Team work makes the dream work" and if you're anything like me, you have dreams stuck inside of you. Your dreams are stuck because you have been numbed to a reality that isn't real. You make a little bit of headway then get stuck again. I hear you! It's not you that's getting in the way. Alcohol prioritizes itself and makes itself number one! It gets the front seat to everything in your life which in turn takes away your dreams, hopes and aspirations. Exactly what it is intended to do.

Let's take a step back though to honour all parts of ourselves and our experiences, and use them to know that we are not alone. To confide in each other, to get through this messy period in our lives, to slash some demons and to come out on the other side as strong, confident and authentic '90s girls!

I'm certain you won't resonate with every single one of my "remember when's", but I'm also certain that you will resonate with at least one or two. I feel like now in my 30s, '90s girls share something special. We love to reminisce about those years, we miss those years, we miss the innocence, we miss the freedom, we definitely miss the boys. It seems like there was always a boy or three that I had a major crush on at all times.

We definitely took those years for granted and surely wished them away. How I just ALWAYS wanted to be 16! Now I would never want to be 16 again. Funny how things change. My 12-year-old daughter is an old soul. She will say, "I wish I could drive." I will tell her not to wish her life away because "one day you will be old with 4 kids, lol" and she says, "I don't wish I was older. I don't want to grow up too fast. I just wish I had a bit more freedom." Fair…

Us '90s girls share such a similar path or story that when we meet another '90s girl in person or on social media there's always an instant connection, and we always have something to talk about, like we are long lost soul sisters.

I think I belong to absolutely every single '90s Facebook page and I share or tag my best friend in more posts than not. Ps the best friend I've been talking about is STILL my best friend to this day. I was 5, she was 8. This year our friendship is 34 years young. It just blows my mind that after all these years "You're still the One."

With that said, amongst my peers who are close friends or who are "friends" on Facebook, I'm seeing a whole generation of '90s kids putting the bottle down for one reason or another. Or some that aren't quite there yet. A few are a couple years into their sobriety and some are still going strong with the partying. It's tough to watch now that I have a clear vision in front of me and I'm not blinded by drunk goggles anymore. I try not to hold judgement because I was that person. OMG! "Brain Wow" how many of my sober friends were judging me over the years?

I think that many of us have just had enough and are just ready to make being sober, trendy – rather than the other way around. I got to a point where I would put my drink down or make sure it wasn't in a picture being taken. I was noticing in how so many pictures of me, I was (again) holding up my glass like I was proud that I was partying and getting wasted.

Hiding the glass from the camera was a little bit of a hint that I had a drinking problem. Now when I see people on the path that I was on, I pray that they too *"Wake Up One Day & Change Their F*cking Minds."*

Growing up as a '90s girl, alcohol was everywhere and easily accessible. It was considered "normal" and "fun" to drink underage and get drunk. It was almost expected of us to drink and party in high school and college. I mean what else was there to do when you lived in a small town?

As we got older, drinking became a big part of socialising and coping with life's stresses. "Beer after work" was a big thing, or "Shots Shots Shots Shots Shots Shots" – You know the song. What about "Oh relax. Just have a glass of wine." If I could only have just one. My husband talked to me last night about drinking again and having a glass of wine at my son's wedding. I guess he truly doesn't get it. I cannot have "just one." It's literally impossible for me. I always drank to get drunk.

After years of drinking and experiencing the consequences of the abuse, many '90s girls are now choosing sobriety. And that's what this book is all about – my journey to becoming sober as a '90s girl and living my life authentically free from the grips of alcohol. It's time to break the stereotype and show the world that being sober is not boring or uncool. We still know how to have fun and live life to the fullest. It's a new way that we need to figure out. We can still go to the hockey games, still cook, still have company over. We can still go for walks (I would drink whiskey when I went for walks).

All of those things are still possible, but now… we just do it without alcohol.

I invite you to stay with me on this journey as I dig into my memory banks and share my experiences with alcohol and how I made my way past it. Where it's not the focal point of my life anymore. It may not be easy for me, but I promise to be honest, raw and real. After all, that's what being a '90s girl is all about – embracing who we are, flaws and all.

This book is for me, you and a whole generation of girls, who are now women who grew up with jelly shoes, bleached hair, smoke pits, skids, flip phones and John Stamos.

I hope you can find comfort in this memoir if you had a shitty childhood and know that it's in the past. Our history may have shaped us but it does not define who we are today.

Maybe you didn't have a shitty childhood but then were introduced to alcohol at a younger age, taking a sip from a parent or older sibling, and continued to, or continue to turn to the bottle as weekends slipped into years. It goes quick!

You began to use it to socialize, then to manage and cope, then because you HAD to, to function because it would help to take away the depression, the anxiety, the introvert in you or whatever excuse you have given yourself to drink.

This book is for my kids, your kids, my husband and yours. To my generation of fellow '90s girls who are trapped in the cycle. To my friends that I have and have yet to meet.

With the right knowledge, support and resources you too can *Wake Up One Day & Change Your F*cking Mind*.

Give yourself a bit of time, probably more time than you are willing or want to give, but trust me it'll be worth it! Don't forget that child inside of you. Healthy, fun, rambunctious, playful. She was all of those things without booze. You are still that little girl just with bigger responsibilities. You can do it now without alcohol just like you did back then.

CHAPTER 3

Who Am I Without Jungle Juice?

January 18, 2023 (my last drink was January 15th)

The age-old questions: Who am I? Why am I here? I certainly have no idea why I'm here or why any of us are here. To love unconditionally? To teach kindness, to care for the earth and others? To be movers of things. Lol. Do you ever find yourself just moving things around? Your kids, stuff in your house? Just mundanely moving things from one place to another? I do often and catch myself thinking, "There's got to be more to life than this." That's what my husband John and I think our purpose is sometimes. As the owners of a landscaping company – moving rocks from here to there, pushing dirt around, lifting thatch up and putting it in bags – taking it to the dump. What do we do when we clean the house? Literally just move things from one location to the next. For sake of context John and I are not legally married but we call each other husband and wife.

Well, that's super boring, mundane, monotonous. Might as well jazz it up with some liquid inhibition, excitement. Why is life so boring? Wake up, go to work, make money, clean and do it all again. No wonder I'm an alcoholic.

Now don't get me wrong. I'm generally a happy person. In public, or on the phone. I'm very bubbly, and have a huge smile on my face. John calls me out on it all the time. "You are so nice to everyone, but those closest to you, especially me – you're such a bitch." I have a PHENOMENAL customer service, fake it til' you make it voice. In private, I like to keep things private. I don't like to share things with others. Why do I have this front? Why can't I be happy within my home unless I'm drinking? I told my therapist that I like to drink so that I can let loose and dance to nineties songs on full blast, to actually FEEL emotional songs. I cry.

If I'm not wasted, music is generally just noise.

As I go through this sobering time, I'm learning a LOT about myself and the effects of alcohol on the body – MY body. I have been abusing myself with a carcinogenic for so long. I'm becoming cancerous to those around me. I pray to the good Lord that it's not too late and I don't have physical cancer but emotionally I'm a tumor to my family.

It's weird because I am a mom, I am a wife, I am a provider. I am all these things and get shrouded all the time from my husband for being a shitty person and a shitty wife but he still wants to be around me. If I'm so shitty then what's the catch?

It's really a tough place to be in. I'm shitty when I'm sober because I'm depressed (from years of alcohol abuse) then I'm shitty when I'm drunk… well… not at the beginning but I hit my point where I'm so far gone that I don't even want to be around me. No wonder John doesn't want to be around me either. I'm an alcoholic and no one likes an alcoholic when they are lost in their other reality.

Are you like me? Do you have a switch that goes off when you are drinking? I never know which version of me is going to come out when I've had too many. It's either emotional, loud and fun or emotional, loud, angry, combative and a suicidal destructive disaster. I haven't figured out a rhyme or reason to who I become. It doesn't matter what I'm drinking. Wine is my "go to" and both characters come out when I drink wine.

I'M AN ALCOHOLIC

How long do I have to use this term for? I'm four days sober now and I'm not thinking about booze, I don't want to drink. I'm definitely detoxing. So if we aren't practicing something how can we label ourselves as that? I was a personal trainer for 15 years. It was part of my identity – practicing fitness every single day. That would certainly be weird if I called myself a personal trainer today, wouldn't it? Because I'm not.

In five years (provided I stay sober) do I say I'm an alcoholic? I'm in recovery? Can't we just stop the labelling? "I used to love to drink until I didn't. That was a past life and I just choose not to drink now." I like that so much better. I didn't have a problem when I was drinking, calling myself an alcoholic. I would joke about it with my friends and family. John would ask if I was ever going to quit drinking, my response was always, "No, I'm an alcoholic, it's in my blood." Literally!

The term or realization that I am an alcoholic has only become a part of my vocabulary in the past two years or so. I guess when you do something for so long it becomes a part of your identity. Took me long enough to figure it out.

Then the jokes about it started coming out, and being an alcoholic is normalized and laughed about.

I know I come from a long line of boozers. I just accepted it as part of me.

Here you go 12 steps… Can you hear me? "I'm an Alcoholic."

I want to STOP saying that now!

If this has been part of me as a masked identity for so many years with such a negative connotation – I think it's time to change the narrative. I think it's time to grow up. Maybe grow up isn't the right word, let's go with being reborn. "They" always say – it's never too late to change. Let's give er a go.

How do we rephrase this? I was an alcoholic? I'm in recovery? I'm sober? Do I have to give myself a title like it's a job? I don't think so, although it is important to highlight that alcohol is no longer going to be a part of my life.

This is my new life and I'm just going to say for now (this may change) that I'm just Challaine and I'm going to live *Authentically Free.* New tattoo idea? ;)

INTUITION

Fuck! I knew it was coming. This always happens. That damn intuition. Change – I can feel it approaching me like a freight train. It happens every few years. I never know what the change is but I feel it. It's always some huge life intervention that I do to myself. I get really comfortable in my life (or maybe uncomfortable) then this wave of change creeps up.

I knew a huge change was coming a couple of months ago when I told John, "I'm not your wife on this work trip." I wanted to work on myself, just plug into my audibles, tune out and work.

Thank you Mel Robbins for setting the stage to propel me in the trajectory of my new life. It's time to get unsticky. I dove into her books and podcasts relentlessly. With her support, detoxing and moving through my process has been easier. Unbeknownst to her, she was a major supporter for me. She has been my north star.

We were working on Vancouver Island and I was just miserable. Wanting all of these things for myself. To grow my other business, to start journaling, to be at home with my babies, to finish some online courses that I signed up and paid for.

Our trip was short and we were home for a week. I didn't put anything into motion that I wanted to. I literally just drank my face off for a week. Puked a couple times – at least my house was clean though. I justified getting wasted as long as I was productive. At least that way my kids wouldn't see their mother wasted on the couch, just wasted cleaning. That was okay, wasn't it? I thought so!

Hindsight is 20/20, I suppose, and life is what happens to you when you're busy making other plans. The plans I was making and the life I was leading was not one to be proud of. Sure I'm now the owner of a 1.2 million dollar house but now I'm 1.7 million dollars in debt (damn interest rates). That's a discussion for another time. Actually no it's not. I fucking hate politics!

CHAOS IS I

Few people know the depth of the chaos that was surrounding my life.

I've always been told …

"You're so strong."

"How do you do it? You are amazing."

"You are an inspiration."

"You are such a great mom."

"You are so smart."

To be honest, I have no fucking clue but I was fucking wasted while being that person you saw.

It's time to get real with myself, for myself, my children, my relationship with my partner, my health, my longevity. I want to be a Gram one day. I want to hopefully have my fifth and final child and watch them all grow up and have children of their own.

Who am I without alcohol? I don't know but I think we're going to find out together.

So, thank you for taking this journey with me as I unpack, unravel and begin to reveal who I am at my core without being shadowed by the smooth sweet taste of Jungle Juice.

I hope you can find some solace in knowing that if you feel fucked up like I have been feeling, it's not YOU, it's the poison doing exactly what it's intending to do… Inhibit your ability to think clearly, love deeply, behave properly and be your true authentic self.

WHY NOW

It's been over 20 years. Haven't you had enough? You're fat, you're frumpy, you can't think straight, you have goals that you aren't reaching. This… (journaling) being one of them, finishing your Interior Design course, your Real Estate course. Blaming others and circumstances for not writing. Just get to it.

Stop making excuses! You've had all this time to drink – you could have spent it studying! Hours and hours of drinking time. You could be selling million-dollar mansions by now. I was literally spending 12 hours a day drinking. Starting at about 3pm and going until about 2-3am. *Brain Wow* – I made drinking a full-time job. Do you ever work too much in your full-time job and are completely exhausted mentally and physically? Well, that's where I'm at now. The stress of working overtime has caught up with me. Fighting with my co-workers (family), not reaching deadlines (goals), not clocking in on time or at all some days (sleeping my days away, frozen and unable to move).

You have so much in you that is important to get out. You are literally just drowning everything with booze, you are drowning your soul. You HAVE drowned your soul. You are dead inside because poison kills. Your body is strong (well, it was), but your emotions are soft, so they are going to go first. You are gone, Challaine. Do you even know who you are without alcohol? Probably not because since you were 18 – drunk is all you have known. Before that you were in high school as an awkward teenager. You went from that awkward teenager to this in 20 years and were wasted the whole time. Congrats though for not drinking when you were pregnant with your four beautiful children.

<u>WHAT EXACTLY IS ALCOHOL?</u>

This is where we get sucked in. Brands creating "low cal", "gluten free", "zero carbs", "A wine a day keeps the doctor away" beverages. It's simple messages like this that allow us to justify to ourselves, drinking their products. Have you ever seen a bottle of booze that says, "Drink me, I'm Ethanol?" No, of course not. Many of us can relate to ethanol at the gas pumps. So, obviously "low cal" is going to look much better on the packaging.

"The alcohol in drinks is called ethanol (ethyl alcohol). It is made when yeast ferments the sugars in grains, fruits and vegetables. For example, wine is made from the sugar in grapes and vodka is made from the sugar in potatoes" according to health.gov.au.

That seems safe and reasonable enough. Right?

Let's dig a little deeper...

WHAT IS ETHYL ALCOHOL?

"Ethanol is a volatile, flammable, colorless liquid with a characteristic wine-like odor and pungent taste. It is a psychoactive recreational drug, and the active ingredient in alcoholic drinks," according to Wikipedia.

KEEP GOING...

"Ethanol is a clear, colorless liquid rapidly absorbed from the gastrointestinal tract and distributed throughout the body. It has bactericidal activity and is used often as a topical disinfectant. It is widely used as a solvent and preservative in pharmaceutical preparations as well as serving as the primary ingredient in alcoholic beverages. Indeed, ethanol has widespread use as a solvent of substances intended for human contact or consumption, including scents, flavorings, colorings, and medicines. Ethanol has a depressive effect on the central nervous system and because of its psychoactive effects, it is considered a drug. Ethanol has a complex mode of action and affects multiple systems in the brain, most notably it acts as an agonist to the **GABA** receptors. Death from ethanol consumption is possible when blood alcohol level reaches 0.4%. A blood level of 0.5% or more is commonly fatal. Levels of even less than 0.1% can cause intoxication, with unconsciousness often occurring at 0.3-0.4 %. Ethanol is metabolized by the body as an energy-providing carbohydrate nutrient, as it metabolizes into **acetyl CoA**, an intermediate common with **glucose** metabolism, that can be used for energy in the **citric acid** cycle or for biosynthesis. Ethanol within the human body is converted into **acetaldehyde** by alcohol dehydrogenase and then into **acetic acid** by **acetaldehyde** dehydrogenase. The product of the first step of this breakdown, **acetaldehyde**, is more toxic than ethanol. **Acetaldehyde** is linked to most of the clinical effects of alcohol. It has been shown to increase the risk of developing cirrhosis of the liver,[77] multiple forms of cancer, and alcoholism. Industrially, ethanol is produced both as a petrochemical, through the hydration of **ethylene**, and biologically, by fermenting sugars with yeast. Small amounts of ethanol are endogenously produced by gut microflora through anaerobic fermentation. However, most ethanol detected in biofluids and tissues likely comes from consumption of alcoholic beverages."

OYE…. Was that hard to comprehend? Well, try the next one on for size.

ONTO THE TOXICITY SUMMARY (*According to PubChem*)
"HUMAN STUDIES: Ethanol is a central nervous system (CNS) depressant. It enhances the inhibitory effects of **gamma-aminobutyric acid** (**GABA**) at the **GABA**-A receptor and competitively inhibits the binding of **glycine** at the **N-methyl-d-aspartate** receptor (it disrupts excitatory glutaminergic neurotransmission). Ethanol also stimulates release of other inhibitory neurotransmitters, such as **dopamine** and **serotonin**. The most common clinical signs of ethanol toxicosis are ataxia, lethargy, vomiting, and recumbency. In more severe cases, hypothermia, disorientation, vocalization, hypotension, tremors, tachycardia, acidosis, diarrhea, respiratory depression, coma, seizures, and death may occur. Alcohol is directly irritating to the stomach and causes vomiting. High ethanol blood levels also stimulate emesis. The concern with vomiting during intoxication is that with high blood ethanol concentrations, the muscles that control the epiglottis become slow to react or even paralyzed. This increases the risk for aspiration. Ethanol intoxication reduces peripheral **oxygen** delivery and metabolism and causes mitochondrial oxidative dysfunction, potentially resulting in shock or hypoxia in an acutely intoxicated patient. Hypothermia may result from multiple mechanisms.

3. Who Am I Without Jungle Juice?

Peripheral vasodilation, CNS depression, ethanol interference with the thermoregulator mechanism, and/or impaired behavioral responses to a cold environment all lead to a lowered body temperature."

"Alcohol produces injury to cells by dehydration and precipitation of the cytoplasm or protoplasm. This accounts for its bactericidal and antifungal action. When alcohol is injected in close proximity to nerve tissues, it produces neuritis and nerve degeneration (neurolysis). Ninety to 98% of ethanol that enters the body is completely oxidized. Ethanol is also used as a cosolvent to dissolve many insoluble drugs and to serve as a mild sedative in some medicinal formulations. Ethanol also binds to GABA, glycine, NMDA receptors and modulates their effects. Ethanol is also metabolised by the hepatic enzyme alcohol dehydrogenase.

"Ethanol affects the brain's neurons in several ways. It alters their membranes as well as their ion channels, enzymes, and receptors. Alcohol also binds directly to the receptors for acetylcholine, serotonin, GABA, and the NMDA receptors for glutamate. The sedative effects of ethanol are mediated through binding to GABA receptors and glycine receptors (alpha 1 and alpha 2 subunits). It also inhibits NMDA receptor functioning. In its role as an anti-infective, ethanol acts as an osmolyte or dehydrating agent that disrupts the osmotic balance across cell membranes," according to www.drugbank.com

Oh, man!!! Would have been nice to know this in fucking high school! You know, sort of give me a leg up on what my future would hold. This would have been swell to learn in the four years that I took biology. Seems pretty biological to me? Reading that scares the shit out of me! It should scare the shit out of you too! It's sad because I can relate to so much of that and know most of the symptoms all too well. Two points that stand out for me are "Ethanol is metabolized by the body as an energy-providing carbohydrate nutrient" and "Ethanol has a depressive effect on the central nervous system and because of its psychoactive effects, it is considered a drug." Makes perfect sense! Scientists have discovered that ethanol acts as a product to produce energy. I would always say that booze gives me energy to deal with my life. I guess I got something right there.

But to know I'm a fucking drug addict! I would never in a million years consider myself a drug addict. I knew alcohol was bad in excess but not to the extent of the description above.

Brain Wow moment here – that Ethanol is a central nervous system (CNS) depressant. Well for fuck's sake! Your central nervous system comprises your brain and spinal cord. I mean I'm no doctor but I would like to assume that I can understand pretty basic concepts. Alcohol literally causes depression.

What a vicious cycle we put ourselves in. We drink because we have a shitty or stressed day. After a drink or 3 we get some energy, some happy hormones that release, we start feeling better and start to lose our inhibitions. Then it's like a crash and burn. The toxicity sets in. The depression. We literally drink ourselves into depression. What a horrible concept!

I'm only four days into this whole thing of no booze and to come to realization after realization is comforting, maybe? I feel a little bit of regret. We only know what we know. If I had known better I would have done better, sooner? I think. I hope.

Learning every day. When you learn you grow. I like facts. Those scientific facts that really break down booze is an eye opener for sure.

So, I guess I've hit a period of growth now. Coming of age, I suppose. Kudos to me!

<u>DEPRESSED</u>

In my personal experience as an alcoholic, you (as in me) aren't depressed because you are depressed, you are depressed because you've been consuming a depressing poison for over 20 years straight and THAT has made you depressed. Hard to believe something is a depressant when you feel so good when you're doing it.

3. Who Am I Without Jungle Juice?

Oh! But the morning after the night before. Ugh, remember when you were 18 and you worked in the bar and partied until the lights came on at 3am? As long as you were home by 4, could sleep until 7 then be at work for your 9am day job you would be fine! Guess what, dumb ass … You are NOT that person anymore! It literally takes you a whole day to recover. Minimum.

But then… You start to feel "not normal" by day 2, so off to the liquor store to get your jungle juice. Needing booze to feel normal, to give you energy. Getting drunk so you could cook/clean. What a waste. Fix your life already!

So "why do you drink?" "Because I actually enjoy it." This is all I can say when I'm asked this question. It's true I like to drink and feel energized, good, free, excited about life, setting goals and getting shit done. At least I thought I was. What people never ask is: "How long do you drink for?" or "When do you feel the effects of poisoning yourself?"

Yes, I like to drink at the beginning but then I can't stop. I start feeling sick and tired then I don't like to drink anymore.

Drinking is a whole process from start to finish, like clocking into work. You can clock in, get your work done then start to get stressed, tired, irritable, irrational, etc, then you just clock out. So when we talk about our drinking and trying to justify why we drink we need to talk about the whole process from start to finish – not just the fun part. That's why some people struggle to quit drinking because the positive or "fun" of it outweighs the shitty parts. We need to see the process as a whole. A whole work shift and what ACTUALLY happens to you when you "clock in" and "clock out".

You hear people say all the time, "it's to numb the pain." Not for this gal. I don't feel like I have pain to numb. Yes, I have my childhood traumas, my heartbreaks. This is a part of life. I've been journaling since kindergarten and going to therapy since I was 13. My day to day's look pretty put together and I'm a positive person for the most part. I believe in the law of attraction, like attracts like. I believe in positive affirmations.

I believe that you should do unto others as you would want done to you. So I don't walk around as a miserable slew. I truly loved how I felt when I initially started drinking. But because of the depressive effects that alcohol brought as an aftermath, the only way to get out of it was to "re-up" and start the process over again.

I did have an epiphany the other day though. I think subconsciously I drink to feel SOMETHING, anything. At first, it's liberation, freedom, then it's anger, sadness, exhaustion, tears, and, not very often, but a handful of times thinking it would be okay if I died tonight.

The biggest feelings I have are for my kids. I'm literally in love with all four of them. Their beauty, talent and love they project makes me ball sometimes. They are my soul mates. We are connected. I was the same with my dad. He is my soulmate too. Even after a couple of years after his passing. For example, his clock will go off at supper time and my emotions just well up thinking of him.

Aside from my kids and my dad, I'm a pretty factual, hardass who doesn't show emotion to anything else. I would have no problem expressing ANY type of emotion when drinking though. Maybe my soul needed that expression because I can't *actually* be emotionless. Alcohol was the only way to get something out. Does that make sense?

January 15, 2024 – The night I took my last drink, which was only a few days ago (I hardly remember it) but John was saying how I was talking about suicide. I had 1.5 bottles of wine, about half a 26 of Canadian Club whiskey, smoked some weed, and took lorazepam. The pill was so little. I thought: "How many would I have to take to just end it all tonight?"

Why the fuck are you thinking like that? Challaine, you are terrified of death! Well… full circle. It's the booze. The booze has poisoned your soul. There's nothing left in you, and then you fill it with more poison when it's empty. No wonder you are a fucking crazy person. You are literally filling your body to turn you into something you aren't. The dichotomy is that It

3. Who Am I Without Jungle Juice?

HAS become you. Your mind has become the poison you consume.

Booze has its own personality. It's a drug like any other. Challaine, you are out of control. You have spent hundreds of thousands of dollars gambling when drinking. You have spent your family's money gambling when drinking. The amount of cigarettes you have smoked because of guess what??? Drinking. Let's keep going… this is fun. You have slept with people you didn't even know when drinking you have done drugs when drinking. You've cheated. You've kissed girls, even though you are as straight as an arrow. You have gone to FUCKING JAIL! You even went so far as to puke at the top of the Eiffel Tower. Literally nothing positive has come from you abusing alcohol. Do you get it yet?

They say you are crazy when you start answering your own questions and that insanity is doing the same thing over and over again while expecting different results.

I'm no doctor, but I feel like a self-diagnosis is in order.

Yes! I get it now. It's time to stop. I need a divorce from Jungle Juice. I need to be me without that influence. I need to see who I am, really, truly.

"I Puked On The Top Of The Eiffel Tower" was another title I had for this book as I thought it would definitely make me stand out from the crowd. Well it certainly did on that chilly September evening. Omg, how embarrassing!

That title would have been a great dichotomy description of my life enacted as a metaphor for the highs and lows of my life with alcohol. From the highest points of feeling liberated and carefree. I mean I was in Paris with the love of my life at the time, drinking wine at the top of one of the most iconic landmarks in the world. It should have been the most romantic experience.

It wasn't.

I'm sure he had to carry my drunk, sloppy ass back down. I don't remember anything about going to the Eiffel Tower except scouring the park for a vender selling wine so we (mostly I) could get as drunk as possible before we went to the top and had to pay premium prices per glass (which was probably the same amount for a bottle at the bottom). Whatever my mind could conjure up to get and keep a buzz going for as long as possible in the most cost-effective way. The only other thing I remember was quietly puking behind the garbage can and feeling a sense of pride knowing that I did it so eloquently and discreetly.

That was certainly a low point in my life. In hindsight though, right? How trashy is that? I suppose I can't truly live out the full regret because I hardly remember it. Maybe that's a good thing?

I know that I am ready to move on from this toxic relationship with alcohol and discover who I truly am.

Let's keep unraveling my story of survival, growth, and self-discovery.

CHAPTER 4
Why Do I Keep Poisoning Myself?

I know what it's like to be healthy. Fuck! I was a successful Personal Trainer for 15 years, one that my clients looked up to. I was certified as a Natural Nutritionist. I did all the right things. I ate the right foods.

Nobody knew that I was a drunk. It's true that people never know what goes on behind closed doors.

After working at the gym, I would go home and drink. There were times that I would text my clients the night before, cancelling on them because I knew it would be a late night. What I really knew was that it was going to be a shitty morning. To all those clients: I'm so sorry.

There were mornings at the gym. Not many but I would be hungover and have to cancel my day after the first few clients. I'm pretty sure I puked a few of those days. To all those clients: I'm so sorry.

I'm sorry that I let you down when you came to me for support and guidance. There is no excuse, just heartfelt love sent with a million "I'm sorry's."

I do need to emphasize that it would have been practically impossible for me to drink the way I had been drinking the past year, back then. There was no way that I would drink until 2 am then be up at 4 to train at 5. Never did I put your safety at risk. I promise. It was the past 7 years or so where my drinking really got out of control. I was no longer working as a trainer.

Is Childhood Trauma The Reason I Keep Poisoning Myself?

Childhood trauma? I call bullshit. I've processed my past over and over again. I've definitely spent thousands on therapy. I call bullshit on blaming my past traumas for being 100% to blame today. Do they bury inside of us? Of course they do, but like how long do we need to talk about it for? If the therapy is working then we should be able to let go and let God at some point. By God I'm referring to the universe, the greater power, the creator. I'm referring to whomever or whatever you believe in. If it's a man in the sky, then so be it.

We can begin to recognize that our traumas are in the past and that they may have shaped us into the people we are today but they no longer define us!

I mean, seriously... Am I supposed to blame my drinking on my childhood trauma when I'm 80? I guess anything is possible as I believe the soul doesn't age, just our bodies. With that said though, at this rate I'm definitely not going to make 80...40 feels like a stretch. To think that I could be dead at 40. That's only a year and a half away. I would still have two kids under 5. Without a mother. I had an emotionally absent mother. To be emotionally and physically absent from my children would be the worst case scenario for them. To continue drinking would be to prove that I've chosen alcohol over them.

With the current heart palpitations, the constant consumption of this fake reality, the bad decisions, the wreck I'm sure my organs are in, now going to pills. If haphazardly my insides are okay which would be a miracle then dementia or Alzheimer's is going to get me by 60. I'm sure of it. I can only kill so many brain cells until there's none left. Then I'm literally just a shell of a soulless waste of space.

I've always been a social drinker until I wasn't and really enjoyed drinking by myself. More often than not when I drank I would get out of control and make ridiculous decisions. I would barely wake up in the morning hungover, full of regret

4. Why Do I Keep Poisoning Myself?

and shame. Oh, the regret and the shame along with the disgust and embarrassment. They always pass, but they are literally the worst feelings ever! I rather puke all morning than live inside my head the morning after the night before.

It's weird how the hangovers change as you get older. In my 20s I would wake up, puke for a couple hours, feel like shit eat some crap food, pop a Tylenol (maybe) then head off to work.

Now in my late 30s I can chug water the night before, take an Alka Seltzer and feel like absolute shit in the morning. The am pukes don't happen (cuz' they've likely happened the night before), wake up at 4 am for no reason whatsoever then lie there for hours – like allll the hours of the day doing nothing. A shut out from the world. It feels like the stage right before death. Just counting the hours before it's bedtime. Wishing the day away. Literally counting down until I can start over tomorrow. Too hungover to feel normal, but still contemplating drinking to feel normal.

Again....

I'll do better tomorrow. I'll only have one bottle instead of two. I'll be in bed by 9. Yeah, right, who am I kidding? That's when the "party" of 1 is getting started. Bedtime ends up being between 2-4. John getting pissed cuz I "never know when to shut er down." In my defense, if I have one, I'm either cooking, cleaning, organizing or scrolling social media. Actually nope, no defense. All of those things could have been done sober.

P.S. Here's a little secret: "I'll do better tomorrow" never happens.

Until it does!

What is the addiction to the fights, the emotional outbursts, texting anyone and everyone, regrettable Facebook posts, just being completely emo? It's literally the same thing every single time. Not at first, but it always ends the same way.

THE REAL YOU

They say that "the real you" comes out when you are drinking.

The more I learn about alcohol, what it actually is and how it affects the body and recognize that it is truly a drug – I don't believe it brings out the "real you." It completely changes who the real you is. It alters your physical and mental abilities entirely.

Let's look at it this way. I'll keep it simple.... Where we can relate.

Say you have a glass of orange juice and you add vodka to it. Its name completely changes. It is no longer orange juice. It's now known as a screwdriver. *Brain Wow* moment.

It's pretty simple math if you think about it.

Take the physical molecular being of Challaine, add wine, and you now have someone completely different. The original physical chemistry of Challaine doesn't exist anymore. It's like Challaine 2.0.

Let's take this simple idea and allow for some grace towards ourselves. To all the shit disturbances we have caused, to the ones we have hurt, to the lies we have told, to the stupid posts we have made, to the fights we have gotten into.

Let it go. There's no sense hanging onto any of that anymore, as long as you are ready to do better and move forward. Nothing you do will erase the past but you are only one decision away from a phenomenal future.

I get it, I've done a ton of shitty shit too. What purpose does it serve me to sit in that space? None, absolutely zip and nada.

If you have never heard of the *Serenity Prayer*. Here it is for you. It's a lovely reminder to recite to yourself. Alcoholics Anonymous has been using this religiously so much so it has been coined by AA.

Like I said, this is going to be a learn as we grow, book. I've known about this prayer for years but didn't have any idea that AA took it on. I just found this out.

4. Why Do I Keep Poisoning Myself?

So, here it is. Read it once, then read it again, then again until it resonates with you.

"God grant me the serenity to accept the things I cannot change; Courage to change the things I can; And wisdom to know the difference. Living one day at a time; Enjoying one moment at a time; Accepting hardships as the pathway to peace."

www.lords-prayer-words.com/famous_prayers/god_grant_me_the_serenity.html

Do not let your past consume you anymore. We're done with it. We have to keep on keeping on. Not just for our family but our friends, our pets, our neighbours, our co-workers. If someone matters to you, then guarantee you matter to someone back. You matter!

If you feel that you don't have anyone in your corner. If you have burned all of your bridges, then build a new bridge. It doesn't have to be made of steel – popsicle sticks will do for now.

There's always one person on this planet that's rooting for you ;). Remember, I said I was here to hold your hand as we navigate this journey together. We're only on chapter 4 hunnie, and I haven't let go.

I'll be that one person.

MY VICIOUS CYCLES

I am using this memoir as a means to try to understand why I am the way that I am. What it comes down to – is that I am healing. I don't feel like I'm healing from childhood trauma. I feel like I'm healing from suppressing who I am. From masking my authentic self. Healing from the physical damage that I have done.

It's time to take care of my body, my mind and find my soul. You too, k?

Round and round the merry go round.

That's what it's like with alcohol.

Let's be honest... There's nothing fun about spinning around in a circle until you are ready to puke. The thrill of it is being with your friends, figuring out who's going to go first, "I will if you will. You go first." The rise in adrenaline as you start to go faster and faster, one more big spin until you know you have hit your point..... You slide off, get up, try to walk and then puke or get pissed at your friend for going too fast. A fight starts: "you told me to go faster." "No I didn't, I said don't go so fast." Friends off. All because of a misunderstanding.

It's the same with booze. Get ready for a night out (or in), it's fun and exciting, the drinks start to pour. "Shots, shots, shots." "I will if you will. You go first." Someone says something just slightly off – a misunderstanding, then BOOM – sometimes an all-out war. Friends off. In my case it usually ended with, "I want a divorce" or "you're a shitty mom." More often than not I would be throwing my engagement rings across the room or into a garbage can. A couple of times in public garbage cans or across parking lots.

My fights were predominantly with a partner, not so much friends...

All because of a little he said/she said? Can you actually remember the exact cause of some of the fights you have had with your spouse/friend while you have been drinking? I can't. But... There were A LOT.

That's a sad fact. In almost seven years of being with John, I'm unable to recall the basis of any one of our heated arguments. I remember some of the events during the arguments. One that stands out was that I came into the bedroom while he was sleeping, we started bickering about something then I tried to get him out of the room and off of "my mattress." I was literally trying to get my KING size mattress out of the door.

Have you ever tried to move a king-sized mattress? With someone else it's fucking hard, but by yourself with a grown man on it? Ridiculous. I'm pretty sure John got that one on video. He's gotten a few good ones of me on video.

There's that shame and regret popping in. There's literally nothing that I can do about it so there's no sense in hanging onto that moment. It happened, it is literally now a part of my story, but it's not my whole story. All of the little stories in my life have brought me here, to share with the world. If I could change my past then I wouldn't be where I am today. I used to always say, "Just because we don't know right now, we always find the answer. More often than not we just don't figure out the answer on our own time. It's not up to us."

We know that everything happens for a reason. When there's something negative going on in your life, you can get so deep as to question your own existence. That's a dark place to be. Although every single time we figure out the answer. It could be later the same day, in a week or for me with the mattress example above... years.

Don't expect the answers you receive to be some huge gargantuan revelation in your life. It could be something so small. Like my mattress situation. If that didn't happen then I wouldn't be able to share it within my story in order to relate to others who may have had ridiculous outbursts similar to mine. For me to remind others to let the past go and to not let it define them and to know that I understand and have been there. They (you) are not alone. That's it, simple...

If someone would have told me years ago that my mattress situation where I was trying to haul John out of the room on it would be a point in a sobriety book in order to help others I would have laughed and thought they were crazy.

IT WAS TIME

It was time that I grew the fuck up. For so long I didn't want to grow the fuck up.

As I always say... You will continue to be taught the same lesson until it is learned. Well... for fuck's sake. Maybe I should listen to my own advice.

For those in the back... Let me say it again:

"You will continue to be taught the same lesson until it is learned!"

Let's break that meaning down.

The same issue, traumatic event, whatever shitty choices or decisions will continue to impact your health or your life until they are recognized, dealt with, changed and finally put to rest. Or if you continue to do the same thing over and over again while getting the same shitty results, then it's time to change the thing(s) that you are doing over and over again in order to get different results.

Brain Wow! It's pretty simple….

Don't want to be hungover? DON'T DRINK.

Don't want to gamble? DON'T DRINK.

Don't want to get into ridiculous arguments with your family for no reason? DON'T DRINK.

Don't want to deal with crippling anxiety the morning after the night before? DON'T DRINK.

Want to save money? DON'T DRINK.

Want to lose weight? DON'T DRINK.

Don't want the shits? DON'T DRINK.

Don't want to look like an emotional disaster on social media? DON'T DRINK.

That is what I am trying to do by writing this memoir I suppose. I am ready to face my demons, to learn from my mistakes and to move forward with my life. I always thought I loved myself unconditionally. I guess that wasn't the case as I continued to poison my personal vessel.

I am more than the person I was when I drank. Challaine was unavailable in more ways than one. Emotionally and cognitively checked out. Times have changed.

I am more than the person who couldn't control her anger or her emotions. I mean I've GOT to be.

In all honesty it was physically feeling like shit all the time and regretting the wasted (no pun intended) days of missing time with my children cuddled up like a shit stain of a human in my bed. My whole body just feeling off, hurting, being exhausted, brain dead-actually.

That was another rock bottom... time. It was time. It's been "time" more than once.

A scary reality. I mean to think about it...I've been drinking since I was 12. That's been a huge part of my identity and social circles. Drinking made me feel free and light, sexy in my younger years. But in reality, it was slowly killing me. It was affecting my relationships, my career, my finances, my self-esteem, and my health. So, why did I keep poisoning myself? Was it just a bad habit? A coping mechanism for my anxiety? Now knowing that the diagnosed depression and anxiety was from the alcohol. Or was there something deeper going on? As much as I want to blame my childhood or past trauma, I have to take responsibility for my own actions and decisions. I chose to drink and I chose to continue drinking despite the negative consequences.

It's time for me to break this vicious cycle and start living my life on my own terms. Not booze's terms. It's time to stop being controlled by alcohol and start taking control of my life. It's time to face my life without relying on alcohol as a crutch.

See what I mean? There was no "rock bottom" for me. It was just time. I'm so grateful that *I Woke Up One Day & Changed My F*cking Mind.*

I'm ready to continue my life story and no longer have the title "alcoholic" attached to it-even though I have only adopted it within the past couple of years – when in reality I've been an alcoholic pretty much my whole adult life. So, I'm taking that first step towards authenticity and I'm not looking back.

Well... actually I will, but as a gentle reminder of the life that I once had is not one that I want moving forward. I don't want me being a drunk to be the legacy that I leave for my beautiful children. I am more than what's in a bottle. I want to be here for them, to teach them, to show them that we can grow and do better. That we don't have to stay stuck in the past. That every day is an opportunity to become a better version of ourselves, but most importantly knowing that I am just one decision, or one second away from exchanging my life for a life I couldn't even imagine existed for myself. You too!

Every day is a new journey, a new adventure, and a new opportunity to discover who I truly am without the influence of alcohol. I am proud to say that after a few short days. At the time of this writing I am only 5 days sober, and I no longer feel the need to "feel something" through drinking. Don't get me wrong. Have I thought about having a drink? Hell, yeah! I've thought about having a drink every day. I've thought about what it will be like going on vacation and not drinking. I've thought about summer and gardening while not drinking – just cuz' I've thought about it though – doesn't mean I'm going to. I just need to keep reminding myself that if history repeats itself then NOTHING good comes from drinking alcohol. I've tried moderation – It's not for me. We definitely don't understand each other. I'm an all or nothing kind gal. So I'm telling alcohol to fuck off and be all into myself to secure a big bright and happy future. I need to start celebrating the little wins. I'm 5 days sober! That's incredible! I went from drinking 10 hours a day to zero hours a day! Good job, Challaine! Keep going!

I will remind myself of the anxiety, the shits, the headaches, the fights, the restless nights, the wasted days, all the shit that doesn't make alcohol worth it anymore. Why did I give it so much credit? Time is the most common commodity that most of us take for granted. I'm done with that and want to be present. I want to go to my kids' sports and not look for a bar that's selling alcohol. I'm not going to be packing it in my water bottle anymore. Mommy wasn't showing up 100%, 100% of the time. It was alcohol or the hangover from alcohol. Not every single time, but definitely more times than I would like to admit. I'm sorry my beautiful children.

I will not allow alcohol to take my experiences with my children away from me anymore. It's had enough of my time and energy.

4. Why Do I Keep Poisoning Myself?

I am finally ready to start facing my life head on and deal with it in a healthy way, without relying on a socially acceptable poison.

I aspire to inspire others and change the narrative and stigma around alcohol. Even if it's just one person. I'm here to be of service to others.

I've been battling demons that I didn't even know I had. Who are these demons? Why do they want to stay with me?

Where does this bad come from? I literally came across something the other day. I'm unable to give credit where credit is due as it is posted all over the internet without any direct source. This has, however, helped me see things a little differently.

Now I'm going to preface this by saying, I did mention in my introduction that I'm not going to preach to you to find God, although I encourage you to remain open to anything especially if being closed minded and your something hasn't been working for you, maybe your something needs to change? Here it is. A conversation between a teacher and student about good and evil.

"Why did God create evil? The answer struck me to the core of my soul!

A professor at the university asked his students the following question:

"Everything that exists was created by God?"

One student bravely answered, "Yes, created by God."

"Did God create everything?" a professor asked.

"Yes, sir," replied the student.

The professor asked, "If God created everything, then God created evil, since it exists. And according to the principle that our deeds define ourselves, then God is evil."

The student became silent after hearing such an answer. The professor was very pleased with himself. He boasted to students for proving once again that faith in God is a myth.

Another student raised his hand and said, "Can I ask you a question, professor?"

"Of course," replied the professor.

A student got up and asked, "Professor, is cold a thing?"

"What kind of question? Of course it exists. Have you ever been cold?"

Students laughed at the young man's question.

The young man answered, "Actually, sir, cold doesn't exist. According to the laws of physics, what we consider cold is actually the absence of heat. A person or object can be studied on whether it has or transmits energy. Absolute zero (-460 degrees Fahrenheit) is a complete absence of heat. All matter becomes inert and unable to react at this temperature. Cold does not exist. We created this word to describe what we feel in the absence of heat."

A student continued, "Professor, does darkness exist?"

"Of course, it exists."

"You're wrong again, sir. Darkness also does not exist. Darkness is actually the absence of light. We can study the light but not the darkness. We can use Newton's prism to spread white light across multiple colors and explore the different wavelengths of each color. You can't measure darkness. A simple ray of light can break into the world of darkness and illuminate it. How can you tell how dark a certain space is? You measure how much light is presented. Isn't it so? Darkness is a term man uses to describe what happens in the absence of light."

In the end, the young man asked the professor, "Sir, does evil exist?"

This time it was uncertain, the professor answered, "Of course, as I said before. We see him every day. Cruelty, numerous crimes and violence throughout the world. These examples are nothing but a manifestation of evil."

To this, the student answered, "Evil does not exist, sir, or at least it does not exist for itself. Evil is simply the absence of God. It is like darkness and cold – a man-made word to describe the absence of God. God did not create evil. Evil is not faith or love, which exist as light and warmth. Evil is the result of the absence of Divine love in the human heart. It's the kind of cold that comes when there is no heat, or the kind of darkness that comes when there's no light."

The student's name was Albert Einstein."

Now that definitely brings up a bit of new insight, doesn't it?

Without getting religious, the focal point is clear that evil is just the absence of love. When we torture ourselves and continually poison ourselves we aren't loving ourselves. It's not that we are evil, it's that we don't feel worthy to love ourselves wholly, truly and unconditionally.

That text was definitely a *Brain Wow* moment for me. Holy shit.

Look how we take our past experiences to deem ourselves unworthy of love, our own personal love. Why do we want to sit in the past and torture ourselves? One way to help dig ourselves out is to give ourselves love, because when there's love, it's impossible for there to be evil.

CHAPTER 5
Fucking Childhood Trauma

I've been seeing therapists since I was twelve. First was a psychologist because I apparently had behaviour issues. Then I started seeing another one some time after I got molested by an old man (our neighbor). I'm sure he's long dead by now. At that time I think he was in his '60s.

My mother didn't believe me. Not sure I need to get into it here, as I've told the story a thousand times. I honestly don't feel that it's relevant in my life anymore. I'VE PROCESSED IT!

Although…

For the sake of this memoir I suppose it's important to share – AGAIN. Now that it's out there. If someone asks or it comes up in conversation I'll just say, "Read my memoir – Chapter 5," lol.

My childhood home.

We had a boarder (someone to rent a room in our house to help pay the mortgage).

Before I go any further with this… I originally had his name in my book. As I go through and do my final read I am removing his name as I don't want it to live on. I didn't want to give him a different name in my book as it just didn't make sense to me.

Alrighty…

We first started getting boarders through our neighbor a few doors down. He worked on the reserve removing shrapnel and clearing military debris from the grounds (at least this was my understanding of what he did and is my memory of it today).

This shithole of a man ended up kind of being a "family friend" I suppose. He would have his coworkers contact my mother to see if she had a room available to rent.

I got to know him as the nice old man down the street. He had a dog that I liked to play with.

One day, he broke his ankle and ended up needing help around his house cleaning and help walking his dog. I was extremely happy to help. I was about 11 or 12.

Shithole paid me about $25/hour. That was HUGE money to a kid in the nineties!

I cleaned his place and walked his dog once a week or so. Fine, no problem.

At that young age, as most girls my age were…. we were OBSESSED with boy bands – especially the Backstreet Boys. I bought every *Bop* magazine I could get my hands on and every other teeny bopper magazine out there.

The internet was just coming out at this point also. We didn't have a computer, but he had one AND a printer. He invited me to stay many times after my "work" to use his computer and print however many images that I wanted of the Backstreet Boys so I could plaster them all over my walls in my bedroom. When I say plastered, I mean plastered! By the end there wasn't even an inch to spare.

I loved going over there as often as I could so that I could keep decorating.

One day after cleaning and printing, he was sitting next to me at the desk and went to a website called persiankitty.com. My first introduction to porn. Again, I was twelve or so. The same age my oldest daughter is now.

I was wearing shorts and he started rubbing my leg. I remember his long disgusting fingernails, scratching across my thigh.

I left.

5. Fucking Childhood Trauma

But I came back… Him showing me porn became a regular thing.

Still printing.

After a day of printing, he was sitting on the sofa and asked me to watch a movie with him. I reluctantly agreed and sat in the armchair to his right. Some time had passed and he asked me to sit beside him. I'm sure I hesitated at first and then I agreed. I'm not sure why? I didn't want to make him mad, maybe? I didn't want to give up my opportunity to print my pictures? I was scared?

I got up then sat down…

Beside him.

He kept asking me to move closer to him.

Hesitant.

Scared.

"No."

I did.

He put his right arm around me and went up my shirt and then under my bra.

I guess 13-year-old titties were all the rage for 60-year-old men. WTF?!

It didn't last long, but it was definitely my last time there.

I went running home, up the stairs to my mother's bedroom. She was always in her bed. Told her what happened and in the most loving way possible…

She.

Didn't.

Believe.

Me.

Bitch.

The neighbour had a girlfriend at the time that this happened.

She had two daughters. I never spoke to them. I couldn't even tell you their names.

I went to the police about what had happened to me because I wanted to make sure that what he did to me didn't happen to them.

We had a court date.

The girls were there in the same courtroom. I do remember the feeling though when I saw them in court and my thought of "Fuck! He got to them too."

He got to them too. I was too late.

Now do I feel guilty about this? I'm sure I've carried subconscious guilt around as I went to the police to protect them. Do I think about it? That I couldn't save them? No, not really. I was thirteen. That's not fair to little Challaine to put that amount of pressure on herself. I don't know what happened to him. I've tried to Google him and nothing comes up. I think I'll call the police to see what information I can find.

Postscript, I did call and I wasn't able to come up with anything without going to the courthouse and having them pull all of the records, which I was advised could take months.

It's amazing the things we hang onto over the years. Thirteen… I was thirteen years old and I decided to hang onto this police report. It has traveled around with me in a little blue and yellow bag with a few of my childhood items, like some stuff from Girl Guides, some crafts from kindergarten. Just little momentos.

What you are about to read is the police report from the incident with this man. My perspective and my mothers. She had to write a testimonial too.

These are words from the soul of a child. No editing has been done here except for names and locations in order to keep its original form and authenticity, including punctuation. This is not to hide him, but as mentioned above – it's to not allow his identity to live on throughout MY book. When you see "…" this is where info has been removed.

5. Fucking Childhood Trauma

FROM THE POLICE REPORT – Dated 03/15 1999 – My version of what happened to me.

Page 1

"To start, his name is "…" and he lives at "…"

I used to go to his house just to use the internet. He had no problem with that. I have known Mr. for about 4 or 5 years. In 1998 I went over to his house frequently to use the computer. Since it was the summer I was wearing shorts and it was like he was taking advantage of that. So he started putting his left hand on my right leg. I didn't pay much attention to it. While that was happening he has a pornographic site on the internet.

Later on in July I asked him if I could come over to use the internet but instead he put a pornographic video on the television. I was sitting on a chair while he was sitting on the couch. He asked me to come and sit beside him, I said 'NO', Then he asked me again, I said 'NO'. Then he said 'For just 5 minutes so I said 'fine'. I sat down and he put his right arm around me and then he put his right hand up my shirt and lifted up my bra and was touching my breast. As soon as he did that I stood up and left And I haven't talked to him since. I choose not to.

Page 2

It was in sometime in 1997 that he had put his hand on my leg while we were on the internet site 'Persian Kitty's'

In the end of June, beginning of July 1998 I went over to use the internet but I guess he decided to watch pornographic videos instead. After he did this I got up and left my stuff there. I had about 25 dollars and a few cents. I left a magazine and a slurpee from the 7-11. I came home and told our Border "…" what happened. When I was done I ran upstairs and Told my mom!

My mother's version of what happened

"Last year, after school was out, Challaine came home from our neighbor "..."...

What I remember her saying was that he had asked her to sit beside him on the couch and when she did he commented on her legs at which time she got up and left promptly. There has been no contact from him since then.

At the time, in 1998, she had been seeing a social worker since fall of 1997 and a psychologist since late fall of 97. I had sought out help from Social Services in spring of 97 due to behavior management problems with Challaine.

At the time of the alleged incident she was infatuated with a boy living at Woods' home, Daryl was sent there due to substance abuse. Challaine met this boy in Jan of '98 and the tension between her and I escalated throughout that year. During the time prior to the alleged incident, foster care for Challaine more respite care for me was not available to us (author's note – BECAUSE I WASN'T A PROBLEM CHILD THAT NEEDED FOSTER CARE). I had been seeing out this help because I have Multiple Sclerosis and the stress brought on due to her stealing from me and lying to me and her involvement with Daryl was, at the time, quite severe. So, when the incident apparently happened I went with Challaine to the psychologist and the social worker and we dealt with her feelings at the time (author's note-. WE dealt with MY feelings?)

I believe that in July of 98 her accusations were an attention seeking maneuver so that "the boarder" – who she and her friends looked up to – could rescue her. Right now (spring '99), again, an attention seeking maneuver to prevent her and I from moving. (Author's note, my mother moved us from Alberta to BC so I would get away from Daryl).

In July of 98, contact with "..." (molester) ceased.

In Aug of 98, "..." – the border-returned to England.

5. Fucking Childhood Trauma

At the time of the alleged incident, Challaine had turned 13 and was showing signs of having trouble separating fact from fiction. She showed no symptoms of abuse in July of '98 (withdrawn, personality change, behavior change) nor did she at any time become tearful or fearful when discussing the alleged incident with either myself, the psychologist or the social worker."

Well… There you have it… A shining example of the mother I will never be. This reaction and behavior from her (in hindsight) has formidably shaped our relationship up until this day.

With all of that said, that was just one instance of my life.

I didn't have a terrible childhood. I don't remember a lot of it. Like I said I mostly remember the shitty things. I was and still am an only child. I had an emotionally absent mother for sure. She has MS and has used that as her excuse for her whole life. She kept me from my dad for reasons unbeknownst to me. When I turned 18, I turned to him, and he was the greatest man I have ever known. How could she keep me from him? Why did she let her issues with him become a part of my experience with him? She robbed me of 18 years with MY dad.

My dad has now passed and I think of him every day. A lot.

He died May 19, 2022. My youngest son was born in October of the same year. The tremendous sadness of losing my dad was absolutely heart wrenching. Trying to grieve while being pregnant was tough. I was prescribed pills to help with the grief. I took a few but couldn't because I didn't want to hurt my baby even though the medication was "safe for pregnancy." No thanks.

I think my pregnancy probably saved me from doing some really stupid shit. Guaranteed I would have drank myself into oblivion. Our time together wasn't enough.

I loved my dad so much! He was my best friend, my hero. He was perfect for me. My mother said he was an alcoholic. I have long lasting memories of my dad drinking a warm Bud. I can't pinpoint a time where I ever saw my dad really wasted. He was a great dad. He was never drunk around me.

I guess since we are talking about my childhood, these are a few of my first memories of when alcohol was involved...

I was living with my mother in our condo in Calgary. My mother was dating a man. He got wasted one night and threw a chair at my mum, towards the dining room buffet/hutch. I couldn't have been much older than 4, because at around 5, she started dating our boarder Jack.

Jack rented a room at our place as he worked on the road as a trucker. They dated for about 20 years. I loved him, and missed him a lot. I wished he would stay. I gave my firstborn son Jack's name as his middle name. NiKylo Jack.

Whenever he got back he always had Crown Royal in his black leather bag. I remember the smell of that bag. Mouthwash, aftershave, excel gum and booze. Twenty-five years later we found out that he never divorced his wife.

He was married the whole time he was dating my mother. I found out from one of his daughters.

Another night that stands out was when my mother had some friends over, and they were all drinking. The husband got really drunk and pushed his wife into our back hall closet and broke it. I'm pretty sure the cops were called that night. I was around 8 or 9 years old.

The final big memory from childhood I have where alcohol was involved was when we were at my Godparents' house in Mississauga Ontario. I was probably 10 or 11? They and my mother were drinking downstairs in the games room. I had gone to bed. In the middle of the night I heard a loud thud. It obviously woke me up. It was my drunk mother on the floor. I had to help her get to the bathroom. I'm sure having MS didn't help, but she was wasted.

I remember.

Where do we stand now?

5. Fucking Childhood Trauma

Good question.

She is certainly one that I have had to set boundaries with in my life. She will still go off in text messages about how I'm not putting my kids' best interests first, how she was such a good mum and how she "made sure" she never drank around me. It's interesting to have the same situation while two different people have different perspectives.

I just simply do not respond to those messages anymore. There is no sense in the continual back and forth. I just rather be kind than right.

We are amicable and chat over messages every other day. She did respond to the message that I sent her which contained the police statements. I did remove some private information from this text. The rest is verbatim.

This is what she had to say…

"I went to court with you. He was deported and we moved to Vancouver Island because I couldn't think of anything more horrific than driving by his residence every day. I didn't know what else to do. I supported you in the only way I knew how. We got professional help, I went to court with you, he got deported and we moved away. That was 30 years ago. I would handle things differently now, of course. If wasn't talked about with anyone, I felt it was my fault, I should have known better. We all do the best we can, if I had known better I would have done better. All I can say now is forgive me and let go of the past, carrying around now serves no purpose. I will go with you if you want to get professional help. I should have done better but I didn't know how. I thought getting him deported because of a sexual encounter, he can never come back to Canada, going to court with you and moving away would have been enough. What else could I have done? We went to counseling & you wanted to end that. I couldn't force you to do anything else. It is still bothering you though it is rearing its ugly head again. Tell me what you want me to do & I will. There isn't a whole lot of time left to work this through, let's just go it and be done with it. This kind of stuff can eat away at you. If you want to go to counselling so you can yell at me I will go let's just get it done, I don't know what else to do with all this unresolved issues you need to help me here and tell me what you want 🖤 😦 🖤 "

I don't think she will ever understand the magnitude and the impact of her not believing me, had on my life.
That's when my soul left hers.
I am grateful for her apology.
My mother loves me very much and my children. She is a great NaNa to them and always sends cards, balloons and gifts on special occasions.
I don't think there are any words left unsaid between her and I.
I have solace in knowing I am strong in my skin now. Because of my past, I am the woman I am today.
She is in her mid 70s and is right… We don't have much time left.
I will do my best and she will do hers. That's all we can ever ask or expect of others.
I love you, Mom.

CHAPTER 6

My First Drink

My first drink was when I was 12. I met a boy on a phone party line. Yep! A sex line.

I remember the number to this day 27-Party! Of course you had to be 18 to call. I was 12 and my best friend, Tori, was 14. To get through all you had to do was say your birthday with the year. Those calculations weren't hard.

We ended up chatting with two brothers on there. Once we got talking privately I said I was 16 to the guy I was into. Daryl.

After probably a few weeks of chatting, we ended up meeting them in person. It was then that I told him I was 12. He told me he was 14. Tori and Daryl's brother didn't really hit it off the way Daryl and I did.

Daryl was such a rebel! There was a hardass mystery to him. He was in group homes and juvie. I felt safe with him for some reason. His bad boy attitude, his rough upbringing. He knew the people in the "hood" where he lived, and they knew him. He wasn't shy about who he was and was always on the ready. I had a sense that he sort of "ran" his community. Although, maybe this wasn't the case and if it wasn't then he sure did fit the role. Come to think of it, I wouldn't be surprised if he had a gun. I'm sure he at least had a knife that he carried with him constantly.

He was tough. I loved him! I remember drinking in the back field by his house for the first time. Whitehorn had a bad rap for being lower income and having an increased crime rate.

There were a lot of drugs and crime in the area. It's in the N.E. I lived in the SW of Calgary. It was a long hike to get there and like fuck my mother would drive me there. If you lived in the south there was zero reason for you to go to the north.

At the time, in order to get there, I had to take the #56 bus from Woodbine to Anderson or Southland train station, hop on the northwest (Brentwood) train, get off downtown Calgary, and then transfer to the NE bound train to Whitehorn. It was probably at least a 1.5 hour trip. As far as my mother knew, I was with Tori at the leisure centre. For the whole day!

The first time I drank was with Daryl – on that back field behind his house. I want to say it was either beer or coolers. He provided it – such a gentleman, haha. Guaranteed he stole it from his mother.

I didn't have enough to get drunk but was definitely "feeling it."

Daryl was my WORLD! I was so infatuated with him. He was my first love. I just wanted to be with him every single second of the day. He was the first guy I would fall asleep on the phone with. He was the first guy to call me "Baby." "No, you hang up first." Neither of us ever wanted to hang up first.

He went to jail a couple of times while we were together. I still have all of his letters that he sent me from there.

My mother wasn't too impressed with the phone calls from jail. Rightfully so, I suppose. At the time, she was the enemy in my mind. Just fuck off and let me life my life. She did anything she could to stop me from seeing him. She eventually won.

Daryl brought booze to my house. I think my mother found it and he was never allowed over again. It wasn't long after that, my mother sold the house and we moved to Courtenay on Vancouver Island.

The animosity that I felt towards her was like no other. Moving me away from my best friend in the whole world and the love of my life crushed me.

6. My First Drink

Post script – As I am doing my final edit for this book May 19, 2024. I just found out that Daryl passed away, April 12, 2023.

I have bizarre emotions reading his obituary. I'm not sure how he passed but one of the condolences shared says "Life led you on a path we did not wish for you – we now wish you ever lasting peace that will set you free."

Rest In Peace, Daryl.

Today also marks the two-year anniversary of my dad's death…

May 23rd. I just talked to someone who knows the details of his passing and unfortunately he was never able to recover from years of alcohol and drug use and wasn't found in time to get help.

I told my mother via text and her response was "not surprising."

You know it may not be surprising to some but it's certainly tragic. The last time I talked to him was quickly on Facebook in 2010. I had no idea that the path we all feared for him was the one he took. I'm saddened that it ended up this way.

Okay, regroup.

MY FIRST PUKE.

Okanagan Cider, probably peach flavoured – 2 litre

Now on the Island, the first time I ever threw up from drinking was with my best island friend, Paloma (I named my second child/first daughter after her). We were about 100 metres from my front door. We both threw up on the pathway. We must have thought it was funny because we took pictures. I still have those pictures in a photo album. I was about 13. There's a *Brain Wow* moment. It's been more than 20 years. As I recount these faint memories, I took my first drink 26 years ago. I'm now 38… 39 in just a few months.

Is Bootlegging still a thing? Back in the day we would just hang outside of the liquor store by the Superstore grocery store off of Ryan road in Courtenay, BC. I can just picture it perfectly.

Omg, how dangerous was that?!!!! Two young girls just hanging out and walking up to random strangers in vehicles (most likely men) asking them for booze. Oh, the naivety of young minds. We are lucky they didn't ask for anything or take anything from us.

My booze experiences started early on. I definitely wasn't of legal age.

Then in high school the big parties started happening. You definitely could not be an attendee of one of these lavish events out in the boonies without Lucky beer, (cuz it was cheap) Smirnoff Ice or the hard shit.

The parties are mostly fuzzy in my mind now. I just remember driving out there with friends and just getting absolutely shitfaced out in the woods. Having sex was definitely part of it in high school. All of us girls dressed like tramps. I'm pretty sure the goal was to get laid or at least to be seen as sexy and to get the boys' attention.

What about those house parties? Like seriously a thing from the movies. Where the fuck were the parents? Didn't the neighbours say anything to the parents?

I'm sorry but if my neighbour's kids had a massive house party, I definitely wouldn't turn a blind eye. So weird looking back.

You know, it's funny… My mother moved me to another province because of Daryl and the negative impact he had on my life and behaviour according to her. Even though I continually encouraged him to stop smoking weed, I didn't actually try pot for the first time until I was in BC – pretty much the weed capital of Canada. So unbeknownst to her, I was out getting high with my new friends.

I was always baked in school. The boys I liked smoked weed. It was a whole vibe. It helped me focus, I guess. I would spend hours in the library studying Biology. I've always loved Biology. Sitting there in the library with my discman listening

6. MY FIRST DRINK

to my rave music, planning trips to Ibiza in my head. I took my first remote personal training course in high school and was eagerly waiting to get back to Calgary so I could go to paramedic school.

Pot was so trendy there. I think because it was readily available and to be honest, I bet you a million bucks that at least 80'% of the parents smoked pot. Having been a teenager to being a parent now, I've looked through both sets of lenses.

So, hear me out. I'm almost 40 now.

I know what my mother was like when I was in high school. Keeping in mind I wasn't raised in a traditional "family." What were the other parents like? They were in their 30s and 40s. How many of them smoked weed? Did drugs? Were alcoholics?

My 30s were filled with copious amounts of alcohol, the occasional cocaine binge, and I did MDMA once. I hated it. It wasn't the same as it was when I was in high school, going to all of the raves and getting high as fuck, hugging your sweaty friends for hours and dancing until the sun came up. I can feel those moments as I write this. It was pure happiness and love. We didn't want to let each other go and face reality. We felt Peace, Love, Unity, and Respect.

P.L.U.R – I had the bracelet – did you?

I still do.

We KNEW that we would all be back together, we would have our eyes and ears out for the next rave and get to do it all again.

Until, well. One day we didn't. Crazy how that happens. Without notice. BOOM! A chapter in your life is over. You don't realize that it's over until you take a step back and be like okay, then, "I guess that was the last time."

I never had any really bad experiences with alcohol that stand out in my mind from when I was a teenager. I didn't drink during the week. We all saved it for the weekends. "Oh my God, is it Friday yet?" Even though we got out of school early on Fridays, it felt like Fridays were the longest day of the week.

Once that last bell rang (let's be honest – most of us skipped last class, ESPECIALLY if it was Gym). But on the rare occasion that we did stay until the end of day, we would strut out to our vehicles. My first one was a white Mustang with blue racing stripes (after I convinced my mother that the Datsun wouldn't be a suitable fit for a teenage girl in high school). I did, however, graduate with a brand new 2002 Dodge Dakota Sport Quad Cab. Oh, how I loved that truck so much. I didn't feel like the "new girl" anymore, that I fit in with the Cher Horowitz' of the bunch. The "I come from money" girls. The business owners' kids. The "Clueless" girls.

My truck was this deep blue color. With my own money, I paid for subs and underbody lights. I don't remember what the "cool" name for those lights are anymore. I had that truck for a couple of years. It got me back to Calgary where I did actually take my paramedics program. My truck was a financed grad present from my mother. Needless to say it got repossessed because she stopped making the payments – by choice. She chose to screw me over and fuck her credit rather than continue for me to have a reliable vehicle in the city.

I was getting ready one night at my house with my boyfriend's sister. We were going out to the bar of course. Then there was a knock at the door. It was like straight out of a TV show where they show up and there's literally nothing that you can do about it but just give them the keys and off they go. However, that's just a quick story of where my mother has fucked me over again in my life.

The popular girls at my high school weren't bitches. When they talked to me it was more like out of sympathy. Super friendly (maybe overly friendly) but they didn't really care about me. They probably knew that they would be in shit at home and lose their luxury privileges if word got back to their parents that they were being rude or unkind.

6. My First Drink

Friday afternoons, rushing home, dumping my bag on the floor "How was your day", "Fine" as per usual, grab a snack and run to the computer, sign into MSN messenger and plan the night – again somehow with none of our parents knowing.

I remember getting ready at home, then getting ready again at either my friend's house or my boyfriend's house to get more ready, lol.

Of course, we were all underage, so we would hang out by the liquor store and get someone to bootleg us some alcohol, or we would call up the one person that we knew who was over 19.

Then it was off to the races and the teenage debauchery began.

Bonfires, loud music out of the back of some country boy's truck with the headlights on. How did we ever get home? Oh!!! I remember a LOT of walking!

Riding the porcelain bus, holding back the butterfly clipped messy updos, hanging out at the convenience store called "Town Pantry."

Back talking the cops. I faintly remember one time my girlfriend showed a cop her ass or something and we didn't get ticketed on one of our ventures home. Oh, man! We were terrible. But were we, though? Not a care in the world. Just had to keep our grades up and we could basically run around whenever we wanted to.

My mother certainly didn't want me home. I tried to be out of there as often as I could. We weren't friends like I am with my oldest daughter. All my mother did was bitch and yell at me. I literally couldn't do anything right in her eyes. I really wish I had better memories of my childhood at home. I try, but they just aren't there. Like I said in the last chapter, my childhood wasn't terrible, but it also wasn't great.

There was too much fucking pressure on me. I didn't have time to be a kid at home.

I survived, though.

CHAPTER 7
The Pain

The brain fog and lack of energy has been a big thing for me, but what other physical issues come up after this long of boozing?

All of the empty calories from the alcohol. Eating so much shitty food. I mostly got my daily value of calories in the form of liquid sugar, rather than from healthy food.

I remember having "popcorn pee" or my piss smelling like a nursing home from being so dehydrated. I've had a couple "injuries" for weeks. One in my hand and one in my hip. They are not getting better AND I broke my toe at Christmas time. I was drunk, of course. In my defense, though, if I have one, it was not because I was drunk that I broke it. Regardless.

I blame my hip and hand on work, but in all honesty it's probably because I'm not fueling myself properly in order to heal. The booze has stripped my body of essential nutrients in order to function and heal properly.

This makes perfect sense as drinking alcohol depletes the body of essential nutrients as it uses up all of those stored nutrients to metabolize the poisonous alcohol.

Boulder Medical Centre states...

"If you consume alcohol regularly and try to stop, you may suffer from anxiety, insomnia, tremors, shakiness, dizziness, and depression. You may also experience impaired cognitive thinking and poor memory.

"Many of the symptoms described above are caused by nutrient deficiencies, particularly the B-complex vitamins, which are especially vulnerable to alcohol use. These vitamins are essential to mental and emotional well-being. The list of B-complex vitamins includes:

- **Vitamin B_1 (thiamin)** – Deficiencies trigger depression and irritability and can cause neurological and cardiac disorders
- **Vitamin B_2 (riboflavin)** – In 1982, an article published in the *British Journal of Psychiatry* reported that every one of 172 successive patients admitted to a British psychiatric hospital for treatment for depression was deficient in B_2
- **Vitamin B_3 (niacin)** – Depletion causes anxiety, depression, apprehension, and fatigue
- **Pantothenic Acid** – Symptoms of deficiency are fatigue, chronic stress, and depression
- **Vitamin B_6 (pyridoxine)** – Deficiencies can disrupt the formation of neurotransmitters
- **Vitamin B_{12}** – Deficiency will cause depression.
- **Folic Acid** – Deficiency is a common cause of depression.

"Deficiencies of other nutrients can also contribute to the negative feelings that frequently lead susceptible individuals toward another alcoholic beverage. These include:

- **Vitamin C** – Continuing deficiency causes chronic depression and fatigue
- **Magnesium** – Symptoms of deficiency include confusion, apathy, loss of appetite, weakness, and insomnia
- **Calcium** – Depletion affects the central nervous system
- **Zinc** – Inadequacies result in apathy, lack of appetite, and lethargy

- **Iron** – Depression is often a symptom of chronic iron deficiency
- **Manganese** – Necessary for proper use of the B-Complex vitamins and Vitamin C
- **Potassium** – Depletion is frequently associated with depression, tearfulness, weakness, and fatigue
- **Chromium** – Enhances glucose uptake into cells. A deficiency can cause hypoglycemia
- **Omega 3 EFA** – In adults, skin disorders and anemia develops as a consequence of EFA deficiency"

My therapist asked me the other day if I've been to the doctor. Nope. I have not. I wouldn't want to see what's on my panel.

But here's the thing.

We are told that alcohol is a downer or a depressant.

Brain Wow moment coming right up. Hear me out… This just hit me as I write this.

I could never understand it because I always felt "great" while drinking. The morning after the night before is always terrible, sure…

But here we go:

The crippling depression is a side effect of alcohol abuse! I always equated it being a depressant to "it makes you depressed when you are drinking." I was like, "Well that's not how it is for me. In the moment, I feel awesome." Well dumbass…You. Were. Wrong.

Depression creeps up and rears its ugly head during the day. I, Challaine, am not depressed. Wasted Challaine plants seeds of depression, anxiety, guilt in "sober" Challaine to deal with, which is absolutely impossible to do on my own. Most people can't deal with depression on their own.

Full circle, here we go. … How do we deal with the depression? Take pills, do drugs, of course, OR start drinking again cuz it makes us feel better – poof! The depression is gone. It's such a gnarly vicious circle.

If depression is a chemical imbalance – well then holy fuck! It makes sense. The alcohol is chemically imbalancing the brain which in turn you end up with depression.

Woah! Deep breath!

Thank you for allowing me to unpack that! It all just came through me right now as I write.

WHAT ELSE?

What other pain or symptoms do I get from drinking?

Not being able to sleep. ESPECIALLY when I'm hungover. The anxiety and panic even when simply trying to take a nap. I've been consistently getting up in the middle of the night between 3-5am to chug water and just be awake. It's ridiculous.

I would think I could counter the effects of the alcohol by taking an extra strength Tylenol before bed, with an Alka Seltzer and water. Believing that if I did this it would balance out the booze and I'll feel better in the morning.

There was rarely a night where I didn't take a Tylenol before bed. If I didn't it's because I forgot or was too wasted to even take one and just needed to crash…

Hangover days suck. I'd turn off my phone, ignore my kids, ignore my business, ignore life and just toss and turn to documentaries on the TV for a couple of hours. Literally just lying there, barely even thinking – just staring at the back of my eyelids. I would then juuust fall asleep for a few minutes – TV would silence…

"Are You Still Watching?" pops up on the screen.

No! But I was fucking listening to drown out my own thoughts so I could lie here with distraction.

FORGIVENESS

My poor liver, my kidneys, my heart! How could I have been so mean? The one body I get until death do us part. How could I let myself get to that point? Point of actual physical pain.

The awful palpitations in my heart.

Forgiveness, Challaine, forgive yourself. It wasn't you! Remember that. When you get into the guilt, remember that it was the poison that overtook your conscious mind. Your REAL mind and body, your REAL self would never allow that to happen.

The poisoned brain doesn't know how to behave properly. It allows us to lose sight of what's important.

It allows us to shut our children out, ourselves out.

It invites toxicity into our homes.

It invites shame and guilt and then somehow the only thing we think will make it better is to drink more. Really? Is that what we think? Or is it the residual alcohol that is asking for more?

It's a sick, twisted and vicious cycle that seems impossible to break. But guess what? It's NOT impossible!

Each and every day that goes by, we become stronger and more confident in living authentically free. You are taking control of your life now and you have the power to choose! Alcohol is not choosing things for us anymore. In all areas of our lives. It is NOT choosing anymore.

It's not choosing how I spend my money, how I speak, how I sleep, what I eat, who I talk to, what I wear, my bedtime, how I talk to my children, what I write on social media. NOTHING! Alcohol is not choosing anything for me anymore!

Say this out loud, "Alcohol is NOT choosing my life for me anymore."

GRATITUDE

I give thanks for the lessons learned. I wish I would have learned them earlier in my life, but we will continue to make the same mistakes over and over again until those lessons are learned. Why did it take so long?

Did it take so long so that I could truly be immersed in it and have a history with a story to tell so that I'm able to show my strength and resilience to my children? Set the example that they too can overcome anything? Or so that I could help others along their journey through sobriety? You know, I would be happy with either of those scenarios. I've always been one to help where I could. I was a coach for 15 years and I loved it so much! If I get to coach and lead others and build a community because of my journey then I would be so grateful. I am grateful to you, my amazing reader. Thank you for being here with me as I unravel and unpack my life in real time.

Even though they may not see it now, I hope I am showing my children a snippet of what strength is. I want to inspire others to take control of their lives and addictions. Was I addicted? Yep – cuz that's what alcohol does. That's it's job as a professional!

Now that I'm off the jungle juice, there's nothing in me that wants to pick up a glass (or bottle of wine). When alcohol is in you, it's a party of one and to make the party better, you crank up the volume (literally! Like how loud do you listen to your music when you're drinking?). You need to invite more to the party so alcohol always wants more alcohol.

Remember… It's NOT you, it's the booze.

You may be like me and not have an actual "rock bottom" and just made the decision to quit. For me it was just time. Mentally, physically, emotionally, financially, it just could not be a part of my life anymore. Enough time has passed in my life that there's NO WAY I could keep letting time pass me by because I was spending it with booze to my lips. Too many days and opportunities have been missed because I chose alcohol over my life.

I want to change the narrative and stigma surrounding alcohol abuse. I'm on my way to a big, bright, prosperous and happy future. I just need to stay focused on my mental health, fulfilling my own dharma and occupying my time with things that grow my brain, not kill it.

Remembering to be present in each moment and not let alcohol take that away from me anymore. It has already taken enough time and energy, I'm not allowing it to take any more. I'm not!

Are you coming to some realizations, as I am as I write this book? I hope so.

We are taking control of our lives and managing it with healthful decisions, without relying on a socially accepted poison. I'm with you. I've got your hand!

You are a warrior and your story will inspire and help others as I hope mine is. As for those painful childhood memories or even painful memories of guilt and shame in adulthood whether it's around alcohol or not, keep working through them and know that you do not need to carry the weight of your past. There's literally nothing that you can do about it, so why carry that ball and chain everywhere you go? I got a tattoo on this work trip. A chain – broken. I put it on my left forearm because that was my drinking arm. The amount of times I have lifted my arm to put alcohol on my lips is uncounted, although now I'm reminded that when I bring my hand to my lips I am no longer chained by the bottle.

If you continue to tell yourself the same thing over and over again, it will become your reality. So fill your mind with positivity and affirmations – I know it sounds dumb but really what do you have to lose? Lots actually – but things worth losing. Regret, pain, anxiety, depression, weight, anger, hate, etc.

What do you have to gain? A whole new future! Now doesn't this sound great? It sure does to me… So let's go!

Start to change your reality with words and actions. The law of attraction works whether you think it's hocus-pocus bullshit or not. Like attracts like.

Start attracting love, discipline, commitment to your health, abundance and freedom from the jungle juice. Even if you don't believe it yet, fake it until you make it. The universe doesn't know any difference.

You are not in jail. You've served your sentence. You are free.

I want you to repeat this until it is your reality, "I've served my sentence. I am free from the grips of alcohol."

"I AM FREE."

CHAPTER 8
What Do I Do Now?

So, now what? What do you want to do with your life?

Like really? Well, I've always wanted to write a book. Maybe this will be it? How me being fucked up can help someone else? With all of those negative and shitty ego driven things I mentioned I did when I was drunk, I am actually a good person, who tries to do good deeds, and tries to be of service to others.

I've always been a writer. The first time I started writing was in kindergarten. I had a little pink journal. I can smell the old pages as I think about it. I actually still have all of my journals. I've always held onto my physical memories. After getting a brain scan I was diagnosed in my early twenties with an "undiagnosed learning disability." Sounds stupid, I know. I feel stupid writing that. However, that was what came back for me though. It helped me to put together a few pieces of my life and a few things started to make sense… My journaling practice, collecting memories, constantly taking pictures and scrapbooking. In grade school I was a phenomenal student when it came to the work. The exams though, I just could not retain any information for the exams.

So, who am I? Why should you keep reading this book? Chances are you're fucked up too. Maybe you aren't but why in the hell would you pick up a book titled *"It Wasn't Jail That Was My Rock Bottom It Was Time?"* Postscript… this was another title in the running.

Amazing how many book titles I've come up with throughout this process. I told you that we are literally going through this process together and that you are getting it in real time.

I will get into really going "through" the motions later on.

The title may change but for now it seems to work.

I don't think I have lived a life too out of the ordinary but looking back it certainly centered around alcohol – from my earliest memories. That makes me sad but it has brought me to here for which I am grateful. I am grateful for the lessons so now I can and will do better in my life.

I have 4 kids, the first two I'm sure I have fucked them up as they have seen the cops at the house, one saw me get arrested, and they have both seen me yelling and screaming like a an insane maniac.

PaLoma saw me stumbling in my bathroom the other night and laughed at me. Yep, just last week. She's twelve. The babies are two and one. Maybe they are my chance to start over, my chance for redemption on this wrecking ball? I hope I can give them better memories than the bigs. I'm sorry NiK and Loma. I guess it's true that people aren't ready to change until THEY are ready to change. I just love the old saying, "When the student is ready, the teacher will appear."

I surrender.

CHAPTER 9
Rock Bottom

So I mentioned that going to jail wasn't my rock bottom. It should have been.

I got day-wasted with an ex and we just started fighting… I lost my shit on him and physically assaulted him.

The cops were called and they cuffed me and dragged me out to the cruiser without my shoes on. The tops of my feet scraping along the stairs on the way down. I had marks for months to remind me what I fucking idiot I was.

This was probably 2017 or so. By the good graces of the universe, I didn't get a record, charged or do jail time. Just the one night in the drunk tank. I definitely deserved it.

Basically it was a first time offence and I got away with, "She's a good mom who got wasted and lost her shit." I am SO grateful that nothing serious (legally) came of that and that I didn't actually do time, just time on a bruised ego and of course I blew up my relationship.

My actions towards the love of my life did in fact dissolve the relationship. That's a difficult event to return from and continue to be in a "happy marriage." The million I'm sorry's didn't matter. Of course they didn't, because they were intertwined with me cheating on him when I was drunk.

We used to go to this bar called Cowboys and would drink and dance for hours together. There was a professional country dancer there who would spin and flip the girls around. He was there every night. I was one of those girls. One night, I went to the bar without my ex and I was sitting with this dancer. We started kissing.

I got a tap on my shoulder and it was my ex. I yelled at him for showing up!

Can you believe that? I was mad at my person for catching me cheating on him. As I write this, I feel absolutely ridiculous. I definitely wasn't sober when it happened. An excuse? Absolutely not but it just goes to prove, once again the negative impact that alcohol has on our personal relationships. If I wasn't drinking, I wouldn't have assaulted him nor would I have kissed another guy.

That kiss was the only time I ever cheated on him.

My punishment for the assault was twelve weeks (maybe it was more like twenty) of all women's counselling. I probably should have stayed. The counseling wasn't to get sober. It was just to talk shit out with other crazies about life.

My punishment for the cheating was that he left me. Not only did he leave me but he left my children who absolutely loved him and called him DaDa. Rightfully so. I don't blame him.

Because I drank two times I lost a relationship, got arrested and my children lost the most loving positive role model in their lives.

After that I ended up going to a wedding in Mexico. He was supposed to come with me. He didn't. I'm definitely not surprised. He did, however, stay at the house to watch the kids.

The sober me couldn't believe what I had done, wishing I could just erase it. He didn't deserve that, neither did my kids.

I was so committed to him while I was gone. I kept the ring on that he gave me. I didn't hang out with other guys. I barely talked to anyone. I made sure that he knew it!

After a five-month separation he did end up moving back in and it was absolutely amazing. It was like a dream come true having him come home. We needed the break for sure. I did a lot of healing in the time that he was gone. I got my poop in a group, as I like to say.

9. Rock Bottom

This was one of the times that the amazing author and spiritual leader Dr. Wayne Dyer showed up in my life. To help me get through the thoughts, motions and the reality of what I had done. He helped me take responsibility for my actions and to teach me about my ego and to give me the confidence to know that I would be okay, even though my heart was shattered in a million pieces.

I would definitely consider those two instances and the impact they had on my life being some rock bottoms. Still wasn't enough to quit drinking.

Fast forward to 2017 when my ex and I were permanently separated. John and I got together. Dating John was fun, exciting, different. He was a breath of fresh air. I felt wild and free with him. I liked his friends and they liked me. My relationship with John started as a work one and then we just became inseparable. We also couldn't separate the alcohol, cocaine, MDMA and gambling. It was so much fun (at first) then as the years went on it just became disastrous. The partying turned into a routine and habit. There were nights where the cops would show up because the fights that we got into were so out of control. I'm grateful that we were never physical with each other during the heat of our arguments.

The gambling was the worst it had ever been for me in my life with John. We loved to gamble so much that we got tattoos of horseshoes on us. At first the gambling was fun and profitable, if you can believe that, but by the end of it we were tens of thousands of dollars in debt.

We would usually start our nights off at home drinking wine and Crown Royal on the porch smoking a ridiculous amount of cigarettes. Boredom would then set in and one of us would get "the itch" which would convince the other one that they had the "itch" too.

The "itch" to go hit buttons on the VLT's at the local pub. We enjoyed going to Bogey's. The people were nice, and the drinks flowed. We became regulars like so many others.

Before we would go out we would always say, "Only $400." We both knew that was a lie. Never in the history of ever would we only spend $400.

That $400 quickly turned into $3,000-$4,000 every single night that we went out.

Because we had been pre-drinking before we got there all inhibitions were gone and it's like money didn't actually have a value. That we could just make it up "tomorrow."

After a couple years of hanging out at Bogey's pretty much every single night, we started going to the casino, and I started going to the casino by myself too. I would always say "You chase the wins and you chase the losses." What I mean by this is that if I would win $10,000 in a night I would chase that high and try to win more. If I would lose $10,000 in a night I would chase that loss the next night to try and recuperate. It was an absolutely terrible and vicious cycle. A $10,000 loss turned into over $500,000 pretty quick over the few short years.

Naturally, I would be absolutely wasted to be spending that kind of money. One spin would start out at $25 and go all the way up to $250! I'm in shock as I relive this. I can remember sitting there with my spritzed wine, a stack of cash that I had pulled from my credit card and just hitting the button. Sometimes it would take 15 seconds to blow $1,000.

I really enjoyed going to the casino by myself. I loved the ladies who worked there, and I loved the free booze. I loved being by myself. Being there was like having a timeout from life. Adult video games… I loved winning. I hated losing, but the thrill was in chasing the win.

Some nights would get really heated with John and I at the casino and we would end up leaving separately. There were many of those nights that I wouldn't even go home. I would just taxi myself to a hotel and crash. There is a specific hotel in town that I would go to. We called it "The Dungeon" because it had a basement VLT bar. When I would come strolling in by myself to get a room I would get the "drunk mom discount." Yep! I weaseled my way into getting a lower price by getting

9. Rock Bottom

them to give me the "drunk mom discount", which is obviously totally made up – by me. That is just so incredibly dumb.

It didn't matter if it was in a hotel or in my own house, waking up and dealing with John, the hangover, the financial loss, the anxiety, the regret and depression were a combination of feelings that I do not recommend for anyone to feel. Then come the thoughts of just ending it. The kids would be better off without me.

No they wouldn't! Who the fuck thinks like this?

I actually drove by Bogey's the other day and it made me think about all of the drunken nights there and at the casino. How I really enjoyed the staff, but not once did anyone working at either place pull me aside and mention that maybe I had a problem. They never stopped serving me. They never mentioned that maybe I should slow down. Nothing, ever!

They did however not have a problem with the ridiculous amount of money that I would tip them. I would tip the cash cage girls at the casino $100 just for cashing a ticket. I understand why they didn't mention anything about my drinking habits, spending, etc. Some nights I would tip out close to $1,000.

Sure, I can appreciate that they are probably trained not to talk to patrons about their habits in regards to drinking or spending, although when a patron is there and talking with you for hours a day can you not as a human see the spiral and offer some compassion and/or concern and maybe help to stop it?

I guess not...

Every night at the casino was another rock bottom.

CHAPTER 10

Consumption At Its Finest

How do I start my new life without the only crutch I've ever known?

I guess this is step one. Write it down and see what comes up.

I'm sitting in a hotel room In Victoria BC. John and I left our $1.2 million home to come here for work. We are house broke and we aren't going to make our mortgage payment for tomorrow.

I was completely hungover yesterday (Jan 16th) on the 14-hour drive. Not with a headache or feeling sick – just brain fog. That's where my hangovers are now – a cloud of fog. Wouldn't it be better to just puke and get on with the day? Nope… I guess when you're old, that's not how it works anymore. It's interesting to see how the hangovers change over the years.

I slept the whole night. Today was rough. I took a picture of myself this morning and I don't look well. My resting bitch face is fully activated, with a couple more chins. She's not happy. To be honest, she's not even there. Her soul is gone. Alcohol won.

I popped an antidepressant. I don't want to succumb to the fact that I'm depressed. I don't think I'm going to take one tomorrow. Let's kick this booze, give my body a chance to breathe, live unclouded, out of the bottle, not drowning, work on things that fulfill me, work on myself, my health.

Give it a couple weeks, maybe, and if you are still feeling empty then try the anti-depressants.

I had a good sleep last night but still felt exhausted when I got up. Felt miserable, felt nothing. I got my nails done (I hate getting my nails done) then got back to the hotel and had a 2 hour nap. I felt worse, I ate a salad today… Felt like I was going to pass out just walking. Laid down again with gut wrenching pains, and then shit my brains out.

Is my body finally ready to purge or is it just so not used to healthy food that it doesn't even know what to do with it? We are here for work but there was a freak snowstorm so we weren't able to work today. Looks like we're hotel bound for a few days. Hidden blessing. I NEED to detox.

Day 3, no booze. How am I feeling today? Still foggy. Still granny pee. My poor kidneys, bladder, liver. I've taken pictures of myself and they are terrible. Who are you? You are unrecognizable. Disgusting.

Still not motivated to do anything. Just write.

Took a lot to hop into the shower today. My last shower was the night of the 15th and I was drunk. I wanted to make sure I was showered before the road trip in the morning.

I showered the night before we left so that I could sleep in longer, knowing I wouldn't be feeling so hot. It's the afternoon of the 18th. Gross.

Maybe I'm not an addict with an addictive personality? Alcohol is an addictive drug. Like cocaine…

I've also referred to cocaine as having one word – "more." I would never just do one line. I always needed more. Just like drinking, I never drank to have a drink. I would drink to get drunk.

I'm grateful that I was never a cocaine addict. When I did it, it would be consumed over a couple of days. Always a bender. Never on its own, always after a night of drinking when I wanted to continue partying.

Why can't I just drink "in moderation"? What does that even look like? Why can't I quit? Why do I have to get drunk, every single time? Because it's a DRUG! It's doing exactly what it's manufactured to do.

10. Consumption At Its Finest

I have learned from my years of being an expert at drinking that having just one isn't for me. If I can learn anything from history then it is definitely a fact that once I have one, one leads to two and two leads to game over and Challaine is off on another planet.

I just get wasted every time, probably because my consumption rate is a glass of wine per half hour or so. Whiskey? A two-shot drink probably every 15 minutes.

I liked to drink while doing stuff around my house. I could never put my drink down and leave the room. It would follow me room to room. If I did put it down and leave to go to the bathroom or go switch the laundry or something I would come back and make sure I had eyes on it before I could move to my next task.

If I couldn't spot it right away, a feeling of panic would ride over me, and my pace would pick up until I would find it. Phew! Okay... Found it – take a sip, probably fill it up with some more booze and spritz it (I usually drank wine with ginger ale).

My glass was always full. Maybe this was a trick I played on myself so I wasn't actually keeping track of how many drinks I had had.

If I'm only filling it by a few ounces at a time, it doesn't seem like a lot. But if I started out with an empty glass everytime and filled up 8-10 times in an evening then it would appear to me to be a lot.

So tricking myself by constantly "topping up" gave me a sense of control of my drinking.

I think I also tricked myself into drinking more by buying boxed wine. It was always exciting to grab the box and feel the weight of it during the night, knowing that there was lots left.

I would be able to save some for the next day and be able to say with pride, "I told you, I didn't drink the whole thing." In my defense, if I even have one. A box is four bottles. I've never drank that much before in one night.

There's been some really fucked up nights while being wasted. I don't have confirmation of this but I believe I was slipped something in my drink while at Bogey's one night. Gambling the night away at the VLT's – getting plastered. Ended up at home. Not even sure how, but I remember the paramedics being in my bedroom.

I ended up in the hospital that night. I always chalk it up to "I know what being drunk is like and THAT was definitely not it. I mean I've definitely been wasted and that was not it, HAHAHA." Well, Challaine, if you weren't drinking you wouldn't have been in that situation.

Even though I have had many nights like the one above that I wish to forget, in the moment they are terrible but somehow I always return to gratitude. Albeit sometimes not right away, but sometimes in my tracks when I'm feeling overwhelmed, gratitude has always been an excellent tool to use when life seems unbearable. It makes me take a step back and step into myself to remind me of how precious life is, how full it is and how there truly is greatness all around me. We are all on borrowed time.

Gratefuls are always a good motivator for me to know that things aren't always as bad as they appear. I remember hearing about gratitude journals in the 90's. From my memory, Oprah started the whole thing for me. I've looked at my grateful journals recently and to be honest... Just keep it simple. We tend to over complicate things. Be fucking grateful for your shoes! Be fucking grateful for the cheese in your fridge! Be fucking grateful the universe gave you another day!

I have been using my grateful practice for many years so they have definitely evolved over the years. You can absolutely start with physical things, then as you keep going you will naturally transition into deeper more soulful ideas. "I am grateful that I have endured my past because it brought me wisdom, acceptance and love for myself", etc....

10. Consumption At Its Finest

<u>*My Gratefuls For Today...*</u>

I'm grateful that I didn't have to work today and that my body can rest from the abuse I have caused. That I can use this hotel room as a cheap detox center.

I'm grateful that we made it though our 14 hour drive safely. So many accidents happen on the Coquihalla Highway. Just a week ago we were here and had to go home because our youngest was sick (he's fine now). I flew and John drove. John was first on scene to a fatal accident and facetimed me. It was absolutely awful (RIP).

I'm grateful that my oldest daughter PaLoma called me tonight before bed, that she respects me as her mother but loves me as her friend.

I'm grateful that NiK asks me to help him with his homework.

I am grateful that I have made the decision to put my health first physically and emotionally. Journaling is cathartic.

I am grateful that I can (hopefully) use my pain and experiences to fulfill my dream of writing a book and in turn help someone else.

CHAPTER 11

Social Celebrities

Why is it such a social norm to drink… all… the… time…? I really hope that with my generation choosing one by one to put the bottle down for good we are setting an example for the next. I love seeing the influx of celebrities getting sober. People in my age range, people I've admired. I'm often shocked to see some of them not boozing. People in high profile social circles battle their addictions in the public eye. We have looked up or admired celebrities for years because of their money, their houses, their clothes and cars.

We need to start admiring celebrities for the good that they do, not just for the goods that they have. I can't imagine having the public watch me crumble while getting DUIs, getting into fights, completely losing it, blacking out, or even just being hungover and trying to go to McDonald's in the morning.

Many of us are unable to relate to celebrities because their lifestyles are just so completely different from ours, although what some have to say about getting sober from drugs or alcohol is helpful in my journey. I can relate to them in a way that doesn't involve fancy cars and crazy amounts of money. Here are a few of the celebrities who I look up to and admire for tackling their own demons and who also *Woke Up One Day & Changed Their Fucking Minds* about alcohol. I hope they have found peace and/or happiness in sobriety.

1. "I didn't get sober to be normal." –Charlie Sheen

2. "The only way to change is to change your behavior every day." –Russell Brand
3. "I used to think a drug addict was someone who lived on the far edges of society. Wild-eyed, shaven-headed and living in a filthy squat. That was until I became one." –Cathryn Kemp
4. "I don't know who I am without drugs. But I don't want to die chasing it anymore. I've had enough." –Kelly Osbourne
5. "Being sober will be a legacy for sure, because you are stopping a generational issue." –Jamie Lee Curtis
6. "Live Fast, Die Young isn't really the goal. Sobriety was a choice." –Miley Cyrus
7. "I realized I had to quit drinking when I woke up on my bathroom floor and couldn't remember how I got there." –Bradley Cooper
8. "Sobriety was the greatest gift I ever gave myself." –Rob Lowe
9. "It took me a long time to realize that if I wanted to be healthy and happy, I had to quit drinking." –Chrissy Teigen
10. "I'm sober today and I'm going to be sober tomorrow, but it truly is just one day at a time….I'm grateful for every day that I wake up sober." –Eminem
11. "I don't need alcohol to have a good time." –Jennifer Lopez
12. "My whole life changed when I decided to get sober." –Matthew Perry
13. "Recovery is an acceptance that your life is in shambles, and you have to change it." –James Taylor
14. "I was drinking to numb my emotions and feelings." –Demi Lovato
15. "This is affecting my work and my ability to show up. That's when it started feeling like a problem…. Sobriety

11. Social Celebrities

doesn't mean that life is perfect. But it does mean that you're better equipped to handle whatever comes your way." –Kat Von D

16. "You have to want to change. You have to use your pain as fuel to make a better life for yourself." –Anthony Hopkins
17. "I realized that I didn't want to wake up feeling like that anymore." –Gerard Butler
18. "The decision to quit drinking was one of the best decisions I ever made." –Zac Efron
19. "I used to think that drugs and alcohol were really useful tools. That was before they became an addiction." –Steven Tyler
20. "I used to think that I couldn't write unless I was under the influence of something. But it turns out that sobriety has opened up a whole new world of creativity for me." –Stephen King
21. "The greatest gift you can give yourself is sobriety." –Robert Downey Jr.
22. "I never thought I could survive without drugs or alcohol. But it turns out that I'm stronger than I ever imagined." –Eric Clapton
23. "I thought that I was invincible. It took hitting rock bottom for me to realize that I wasn't…I was a complete prisoner of my own behavior." –Drew Barrymore
24. "Getting sober is a process, and it takes time. But it's worth it." –Bradley Cooper
25. "Recovery is possible, and it's beautiful." –Kristen Johnston
26. "I wouldn't have a career today if I hadn't gotten sober." –Craig Ferguson
27. "Addiction runs rampant these days, and I just wanted to show people that if I could get through it then

anyone can. And without it, if I didn't sober up, I would not have a family. I would not have a son. I would not have a wife. I don't even know if I'd be alive." –John Stamos

CHAPTER 12
Sobriety... What Does It Actually Mean?

SOBRIETY – What does the word actually mean? Here's Merriam-Webster's definition: "abstaining from drinking alcohol or taking intoxicating drugs; refraining from the use of addictive substances."

What does sobriety mean to me? I don't really know yet. I can't give you the answer. I know that by the end of today I will be three days sober from alcohol. Am I ever going to pick up a drink again? I feel like in this moment – yes, I am, but way down the road.

What if I just get a grip on my drinking? Stop boozing every single day! Don't let it run my world! Drink occasionally – not fucking 50 drinks a week! That's insanity!

I can tell you that writing is keeping me from drinking. Well, actually feeling like shit is keeping me from drinking. John was going to go get his truck into the shop today and to be honest, my first thought was to go to the liquor store attached to the hotel and grab something to drink.

Not a huge urge, more of like a habit urge I suppose. You know what is also keeping me from drinking? The fact that I have read what I have written so far to John. He now knows where my headspace is at, or is not.

I don't want people in my life to adjust their drinking habits, patterns or wants on my account. This is a decision that I am making for myself personally. If I wasn't going to then I wouldn't have made the decision to.

I don't want there to be a big elephant in the room of "Oh Challaine is over, hide the booze." I'm not going to sneak drinks from the bottle, or take someone else's drink.

Choosing to drink has always been a choice. Stopping after I start hasn't been a choice. I know that I cannot have just one. My sober mind makes the conscious decision to have "just one." Once I get going… My sober mind is no longer attached. It doesn't belong to me, and it leaves the physical me, entirely. My body cannot have just one. The intoxicated mind takes over.

I don't want to be that person where everyone walks on eggshells around me, "Oh, Challaine isn't drinking, don't drink in front of her." It's not like that. Why does sobriety have to be a big "thing"?

For someone to not drink is such a huge deal, but if someone does drink it's just the norm. How do we make health and sobriety just the norm? I guess just one person at a time. I'm next in line.

What does sobriety or abstinence mean to you?

No, really… Think about it? Does it have to be all or nothing? What about drinking only on Friday nights? What about drinking only on Vacations? Or only while out for dinner? No alcohol in the house? No drinking around the kids? John asked me what the turning point was for me? I'm not really sure I know the answer to that question. I think it's the culmination of all of it.

March 28, 2024

The weeks before I got sober the bigs were seeing me drink every day, being irrational and confrontational. I was not not sleeping properly. I was having heart palpitations. I was just constantly hung over, throwing up, and my guts were a mess.

I then started taking pills. I've never been a pill popper. I've always been scared of pills. Booze has always been my drug of choice.

12. Sobriety... What Does It Actually Mean?

The day I had my last drink I saw my therapist and she told me to take my antidepressants. I DON'T want to be that person. I think the biggest thing was the feeling of feeling awful. Always. Just the excess of it. I've been drinking daily for months straight. How did I get here?

It's been 72 days and I've committed myself to staying sober forever. I don't want to drink again. I don't like that person. I love myself. Drinking alcohol is not congruent with the life I want to live or lead. I've lived a lifetime with alcohol and it doesn't get better. I will never be different when I drink. I've tried. It doesn't work.

This is part of the journey through sobriety. A couple days in and I was pretty confident that I would have another drink with moderation in mind. Now that I have had some time to heal and grow and build a community that sees me and supports me I don't want to let them (you) down.

I feel that I have been a student for over 20 years learning about alcohol, behaviours, sobriety, recovery, and the temptation. I feel that I am ready to be the teacher and to help others along their journey now. I want to lead others past alcoholism, through sobriety and into living authentically free.

Sobriety means to me....

I'm Free.

Thank you for keeping me accountable!

CHAPTER 13
Christmas House

John and I were living in a rental for about five years. Two years ago we were completely broke (from gambling) and I pulled money off of a credit card to put a lot hold down on a piece of land to build a home in our dream community where we lived.

We had a dream and goal to build in a very specific area in our city. I had no idea how the fuck we were going to do it, but just felt it in my gut that we were. The process of building this house was an absolute nightmare.

I was pregnant with my precious baby boy LunDhyn (never had a drop during my pregnancy). I was newly pregnant when we put the lot hold down. He was born Oct 2, 2022.

A few months after he was born it was back to work and back to booze. I would never drink at work, always after.

Every.

Single.

Night.

It felt like a battle to get the money we needed to make our dreams come true. Let me rephrase that. It was a fucking war! Especially when we both had a severe gambling problem. When one of us would always get the "itch" and then the other would just follow. We're always together. When I say severe gambling problem, I mean like a $10,000/night problem.

"The more you make the more you spend" is entirely accurate for us. We are always chasing money. We make really good money, but we just couldn't seem to keep it.

I do need to clear some things up here though before I keep going… John has been my poison and my rock simultaneously. We have built businesses together, built our home together, are raising two beautiful children together and he took his bonus kids in without question and with an abundance of love.

We got in debt together, partied together, we went down the hole together. Me, 100% worse than him. We were each other's crutches through the brutality. Now we are each other's rocks. John is my person and I know that without a doubt. He is my biggest supporter while also being the devil's advocate. We waltz in a dichotomy of ups and downs. Now they are mostly ups. Like any relationship we definitely push each other's buttons. We continue to seek therapy. He is usually the one who initiates the discussion to book our next session. He's fantastic.

Our relationship is his top priority. I'm his top priority. He always puts us first and treats me like a Queen. He's continued to chase me like he has since day one. He's a romantic to his core. I appreciate him for this life we are building, I appreciate his love and support and I appreciate all of him and his sobriety. John hasn't had one drop since I got sober. Kudos to John!

Will he stay sober? He's not sure but he does know that he doesn't want to start the sober counter again. I can't speak on his sobriety long term, but as for now, he's riding the sober train with me.

We have ALWAYS been a power couple and this journey through sobriety proves that we still are and that we can do anything because we continue to choose each other every single day. He loves me entirely and I love him back.

Okay, so living in the rental… Our lease was up August 2023. Our dream home was ready in May, but we didn't have the down payment, and we also didn't have our personal taxes paid.

We kept pushing with the builder to extend our possession date. She was fine with it once, then again… One more time

13. Christmas House

and we were hooped because she was floating the cost of the build, it was time she got paid.

We moved into my in-laws August 31st. Bless their big hearts. They took John, the four kids, two dogs and myself in without a question. The cat… – yeah, he wasn't welcome but did stay with a lovely family for the time being.

With the uncertainty of the house and living with my in-laws, it was sort of like we were just waiting around, nothing to do, couldn't decorate – I could cook though (with wine of course).

The bigs were sharing a room and the littles were sharing a room. John and I were living in the unfinished basement. My bedroom decor consisted of Airplane parts and Lego boxes with the fresh sound of plumbing to lull us to sleep.

Every day it was work, come home, supper, start drinking, and smoking on the back patio.

Literally every day, many nights until 12-1am.

Get up and do it again.

Knowing we were facing our last extension on the house it was grind time, but we were still short. LOTS!

If we didn't meet the deadline and get the house, we could be sued for the entire cost of the house, lose our original $100,000 that we put into it AND still lose the house. FUCK!

We are so lucky to have such amazing people in our corner. We were able to muster up the rest of the down payment and get our taxes paid. JorDhyn, my 2 year old… She knew we were trying to get this house, and she wanted the house so bad. She called it her "Christmas House."

JorDhyn – Mommy and Daddy got you your Christmas house.

I love you!

CHAPTER 14

An Evolution

Where am I now? Well… I had my last drink a week ago. It is January 22, 2024. Still in a hotel room.

I'm feeling good, motivated (constipated for some reason), excited for my future, getting a grip on my finances.

I'm almost done listening to my second audiobook. The first one was by Annie Grace, *This Naked Mind – Control Alcohol*. What a game changer that book has been for me – and thousands of others I'm sure. Thank you Annie for your help with enabling me to live authentically free.

I'm in my second audio book right now called, *Get Rich Lucky Bitch* by Denise Duffield-Thomas. She is re-awakening me to the power that I hold within myself – that the universe is on my side and that I'm my own block or resistance.

I know all about manifesting the life that I want to live: Vision boards, the law of attraction, being genuinely grateful for all things in my life, giving thanks to the universe for little blessings that we may take for granted.

I've done this before in my life…

My last vision board had four children, being a homeowner, making $10,000/m in income. There was more. I'm sure I still have it and didn't throw it out. I've reached those goals. I maxed out on those goals because of alcohol.

I was in a place so bad that I couldn't even watch the Netflix documentary *Live to Be 100, Secrets Of The Blue Zones*. Knowing that I was a drunk. I just felt guilty. Every time I would see it pop up I was just riddled with guilt knowing that everyone who is on that list and who has something to say definitely isn't living my lifestyle (old lifestyle). I didn't want to listen to it cuz I knew it meant that I would have to give up my daily drinking if I were to listen and implement what they had to say.

I literally chose to poison my body every single day, be scared of death, gain weight, have terrible sleep, crippling anxiety, have mild hallucinations of "things" just appearing out of nowhere and scaring the shit out of me, choosing the bottle over my children (not always but a LOT of the time) and and and – over learning how to live to be 100. That's some fucked up shit right there.

They certainly aren't wrong when they say alcohol kills brain cells. How on God's green earth could I have chosen booze over living?

That's certainly a *Brain Wow* sobering idea.

"I AM A POWERFUL MANIFESTOR"

Back to manifesting…

I was worthy before all of these phenomenal expectations although my mind and body weren't ready to take them on.

How in hell would the universe bless me with more money if I couldn't keep the money that I already had. "Well, Challaine, you can't handle a few thousand dollars, why would we send you more?"

I feel like I'm on the same page with the universe now. That we can work together and harmoniously. That my mind can think clearly and I have a new direction on where I want my life to go.

Holy fuck! Was I ever stuck? Shame on me for what I wasn't consciously aware of. Yea me, for taking action to quit that life and start new – now. It's never too late to be the best version of myself. I can see clearly now without my drunk goggles on.

Committing to sobriety is a profound decision that often leads to personal growth, self-discovery, and positive transformation. Here are some awesome ways that I am experiencing the changes in my life. These gifts are just a by-product of getting sober. I wouldn't trade these for a wasted hangover day ever again.

Check these out.

1. Clarity and Mental Sharpness

Sobriety has gifted me with improved cognitive function and mental clarity. I am able to get a full night's sleep without waking up in a panic, which in turn allows me to think clearly throughout the day and focus on the tasks that I set forth for myself.

2. Emotional Resilience

Sobriety has gifted me the ability to confront and manage my emotions, temper, and attitude. Without relying on alcohol as a coping mechanism, this fosters emotional resilience, providing the ability to navigate my life's challenges with greater strength and stability. I am able to handle my children's needs much better now and have a higher tolerance for them. I am more patient, calm, and understanding.

3. Improved Physical Health

Abstaining from alcohol has contributed to weight loss. Not as much as I would like since I've up'd my evening chips and chocolate game at the moment, but for the most part I am eating better food throughout the day. I am sitting down with my family for supper now. I would typically be wasted and cook these fantastic meals then not eat them. It was more important for me to get to the bottom of the bottle. I could never drink booze and eat at the same time. I am not drowning in liquid empty calories. My kidneys don't hurt. My stomach isn't raw from throwing up. What a gift!

4. Rebuilding Relationships

Sobriety has gifted me the attentiveness that my children deserve. My older children will remember my years of drinking as they were witness to so much. For that I am sorry. My babies though, will not have any memories of their mother being hungover, falling over or tossing aside beautiful days wasting away in bed. John and I continue to attend counseling as it helps to strengthen our relationship. Without the booze we don't fight so aggressively (verbally) anymore There's no more lying. He doesn't resent me anymore for drinking every day. Overall there is so much more calm in my relationships and home.

5. Rediscovery of Identity
Sobriety has gifted me the opportunity to discover my authentic self. Without the influence of alcohol I have been given the opportunity to work on writing. I have been writing for years and always wanted to write a book. Now that I have an ugly and beautiful story to share I am able to write it and get it out to the world.

6. Increased Self-Esteem
Sobriety has gifted me the ability to be more confident in myself and not have this umbrella of guilt hanging over my head for my poor physical and financial decisions. Overcoming the challenges of alcoholism has given me a major sense of accomplishment and pride, enhancing my belief in my ability to overcome obstacles so that I am able to share and help others.

7. Formation of Healthy Habits
Adopting a sober lifestyle has gifted me the development of healthier habits. By all means they aren't perfect but I am always a work in progress. It is rare that I am in bed after 9pm now. I am sleeping phenomenally. I am consistently waking up at 4am without hitting the snooze button and feeling well rested. I no longer spend copious amounts of money on food delivery after a night of drinking.

8. Spiritual Growth

Sobriety is gifting me the ability to look outside of myself and connect to God (Universe, Source, The One). I live in a state of gratitude for my sobriety, my clarity, my surroundings and the lessons I am constantly learning. This doesn't involve organized religion for me but encompasses a deeper connection with myself, nature and a sense of purpose beyond this material world.

9. Increased Productivity

Sobriety has gifted me increased productivity and goal attainment. This book that you are reading has been deep inside me for years. Getting sober is the only way that this is going to come to the surface. With a clear mind and new found focus I am able to pursue personal and professional ambitions with dedication and determination.

10. Community and Support:

Committing to sobriety has gifted me the connection with sober communities and support groups. I have created new social platforms which can be found on my website to connect with other individuals who have gone through or who are going through living authentically free. These networks provide encouragement, understanding, and shared experiences, fostering a sense of belonging and mutual support. People who are sober just have a new zest for life. I'm feeling zesty!

11. Financial Stability

I have been gifted with gaining control of my finances. I no longer spend money on copious amounts of alcohol and take out (between $40-$120 a day if I was drinking at home). I no longer spend an insane amount of money gambling and drinking at the casino or pub. The by-product of that is that I have completely switched my social circle. I no longer hang out with emotional, irrational drunks and my friends don't cost me thousands of dollars. The financial strain I've put myself and my family through because I was selfish is fading in the rearview. Slowly but surely I am redirecting my resources towards personal and financial goals, leading to increased stability and security for myself and my family.

12. Personal Responsibility

Sobriety has gifted me a sense of personal responsibility. I am taking ownership of my actions. I'm attempting to make amends with those whom I have wronged.

Seeking professional help, engaging with support networks, and maintaining a commitment to personal growth are essential elements of a successful and evolving sober lifestyle.

I encourage you to join my online sober community. I have created it for those of us who just *Woke Up One Day & Changed Our F*cking Minds* or really want to but don't know how to get started. Sometimes we just need a little motivation and a kick in the ass. I'm happy to be the one to kick you.

This book was like a massive journal entry for me at first. This book is my heart in words. To share my heart, knowledge and experiences with others who may benefit brings me so much gratitude. I feel like this is an act of service to you my friend. I hope this book inspires you as much as I've been inspired to write it.

Sobriety has gifted me the joy of having YOU in my life!

Thank you!

CHAPTER 15
Authentically Free

I told John today that I am getting a tattoo next week. He was silent. I'm getting resistance from him with this whole "journey" that I'm on. My rebirthed spirituality is making him uncomfortable. I say "rebirthed" because I have been in this connected mindset before in my life where I felt connected to my source. Never though, during my relationship with him. He doesn't know "this" version of his wife.

He said that I've put myself on a pedestal and that I've never put him first in almost seven years. That he's been waiting for me to be his wife – completely.

I was still emotionally attached to my ex Will, when John and I started dating. Will and I broke up at the beginning of May 2017, I met John May 12th, started dating shortly after and we were engaged to be married October 26th of the same year.

Was the emotional attachment fair to John? Absolutely not, but it certainly wasn't intentional. You can't control how you feel for someone. Even though Will and I had separated, that didn't mean that I didn't still have feelings for him. 5 years is a long time to be with someone.

I was, though, completely infatuated with John. He was high energy, attractive, kind, generous, made good money, and was respected amongst the people he worked with. Just like I couldn't control my feelings for my loss of my life with Will, the step dad to my kids. He was the man who changed PaLoma's diapers and who taught NiK how to ride a bike. I couldn't control the new feelings I had for John.

I definitely emotionally cheated on John. He just came into my life so quickly and sort of took over. I had no time to process the break up, breath, or be single…

I only had time to party, I guess.

The beginning of mine and John's relationship started with drinking and partying and gambling (a LOT of gambling). Insert rave scene here, circa 2017. John was definitely a welcomed distraction from Will. Breakups are never easy, especially when you are breaking up your family. I'm never one to just sit in silence and sulk. I have rarely ever been single. My relationships have always gone from one to the next.

I'm sure I have some sort of ADD or something, but don't we all to an extent? I was busy working all day with John, then home to my kids and he would come over, then he just sorta moved in one day.

We went to a Halloween rave on Oct 25th, then on the morning of the 26th as we were really facing "the morning after the night before." A night of booze and MDMA. I wouldn't be surprised if a line or two of blow was in there too.

He proposed.

I said, "Yes."

Our relationship snowballed, and we started building a business that November, then we started talking about building a house. I was then pregnant with our daughter JorDhyn in 2020.

Still emotionally unavailable.

I had JorDhyn in 2021 then got pregnant with my sweet LunDhyn and he was born in 2022. Two babies in 2 years, plus nursing over a year with each one is fucking exhausting.

Still emotionally unavailable

Well, no shit!

During the time of the pregnancies and new babies I just longed to "do me." I wanted to journal. I wanted to scrapbook. My journal is still locked up. Is it so hard to ask for privacy and to just write?

15. Authentically Free

These things would take time, so I just kept pushing them off. One thing I never put off though, was the opportunity to drink. Once those babies were out of me it was smoking, drinking and gambling all over again. After each one I just reverted back to old habits. I literally had zero control over it. Neither did John to be honest.

It would just be a regular night of smoking and drinking on the front porch then one of us would get "the itch." No one more than the other I don't think but this stupid, ridiculous itch to hit the buttons on a VLT. When you win, you WIN but when you lose, you lose. Like I always say, "You chase the wins and you chase the loses." We had some ridiculous nights where we would spend upwards of $10,000 in a single night.

Let me tell you, the morning after the night before. HOLY FUCK! $10,000!!!

All because of alcohol. When you are at the casino and playing with that kind of money and you are drinking, it's like that invincible teenager syndrome comes flooding in and nothing matters.

You get thoughts of "I'm a good person, I have good karma, it's gotta give, I'm such a good tipper, it'll pay out" to "Ah! It's only money, who cares? We're having fun… you only live once." All of that then just complete ignorance when the older kids would call and we'd say we would be home in an hour, then an hour turned into 4. Then we would just ignore their calls "Fuck! Can't we just go out without being disturbed"?

We would come strolling in some nights at 2, 3am with pizza, wings or macaroni bites for them. Purchased as a bribe of sorts I suppose. Actually it's 100% accurate. Feeling guilty for not making supper that night or for being complete assholes and ignoring them.

The crazy fighting that would go on between John and I happened all the time. He's asked for my rings back more times than I can count, whereas I've thrown my rings into the abyss more times than anyone can count.

The cops even got involved a couple times. Like what the hell? (no one ever got hurt or went to jail) they basically babysat us as our emotional drunk asses tried to defend our own selves.

To this day I don't think I could even tell you what we fought about.

I have never wanted to bury myself alive more than the morning after a night at the casino.

I can promise you that all of those thoughts and feeling of "I'm a good person", etc., are a load of crap as you are rolling around hungover, anxious, tired, brain dead, dehydrated, hungry but can't eat cuz you can't move, feeling like a shitty mom cuz you didn't take a child to an activity cuz you physically couldn't.

Having to deal with John the next morning was so annoying. It never went over well.

Then I was guilt ridden because I spent $10,000. The worst part is that it didn't happen just once. The casino didn't happen every night, but we were in a stretch there when we were hitting the local pub every night and spending at least $2-$4K – a NIGHT!

All because of FUCKING ALCOHOL!

Writing all of this makes me so angry. It got to me! It took my money, it took my time – sooo much time away from my kids, it took my health, it took my spirit.

This is interesting to process. We gambled HARD for the entirety of our relationship. When I met John and we would go out to the pub for drinks he would always win on the VLTs. Like thousands at a time. I joined him and won a bit too here and there. We used to say he had a horseshoe up his ass. We believed in the horseshoe bringing us luck so much that we got horseshoes tattooed on us in Mexico. Guess what happened to all that luck? Yea exactly… What luck?

Patterns …. The drinking, gambling and drugs have cycled through my life a few times.

15. Authentically Free

I was with a guy (he still contacts me to this day – 20 years later) who I used to call a "triple threat" – Cocaine, Gambling and Alcohol. Daily.

I would go with him to the pub or casino so he could play and drink after work. It was fun for me because he would feed me money with his wins so I could play a little. By a little, I mean I would maybe play $300-$400/night. I call it "shut me up money." There's nothing more annoying than playing at a machine and having your partner standing over your shoulder, bored just watching and waiting. Like "fuck off." So he would give me "shut me up money" that way I would leave him alone and go play for a few minutes.

Now, back to the past, this bit is a challenge to write because I know my kids will see this, but at the beginning I promised to be honest, raw and real. This is all a part of my past and part of my journey and has shaped me into who I am today so I can live the BEST tomorrow.

As Brene Brown states, *"Owning our story and loving ourselves through that process is the bravest thing we'll ever do."*

So, the first two nights that I ever did cocaine was when I was with my children's father. I had never tried it in high school (at least not that I remember) and I was 22 at that point. We were drinking and just wandering around late at night in our neighbourhood. I got pregnant both times.

What a blessing those times were. A blessing in disguise. If booze wasn't involved, then I wouldn't have done the blow, and then I definitely wouldn't have gotten pregnant with my two beautiful children. Before I got pregnant with my first I had several miscarriages. So many that I started seeing a fertility specialist. Getting pregnant and finally being able to keep the pregnancy was the greatest joy in my life. My son! I finally had my son!

I do need to mention though that cocaine has never been a problem for me in excess. Well that's a lie. It was a problem while I was on it. Benders would last 3 or 4 days then it was over for months, then years and I was just done for good. The thought of it now literally makes me cringe.

It was never something that I got into on the regular. Thank the good Lord for that and for saving me from that kind of life. No seriously, thank you! That could have been a slippery slope for me.

What a fucking past I've had in my adult life. Such nasty patterns. "Why didn't I learn the first time, or the second time or the third or forth?"

Lao Tzu is famously quoted in the Tao Te Ching saying, "When the student is ready the teacher will appear. When the student is truly ready... The teacher will disappear." My interpretation of this is that this famous verse basically means that we will continue to have the same lessons delivered to us until we are finally ready to learn. Once we have learned the lesson there's no more need for teaching and the lesson who is really the teacher disappears. Wow! That's some powerful shit right there.

So what does it mean for me now?

Well...I'm going to say it's been about 20 years of active addiction to alcohol. I always said that I was a "functioning alcoholic" or that "I drink because I actually enjoy it."

I always maintained my jobs, I've built companies, my children have more than they could ever ask for. I did it loud and proud in public but in reality I was doing so much damage. So much damage that I couldn't even see it happening as it was happening. I would chalk it up to a shitty night or bad luck or what other damn excuse I would give myself when in all actuality my shitty nights wouldn't have been shitty without booze.

Well, teachers, I've heard you loud and clear.

My teacher was alcohol. To show me the world I don't want to live in anymore.

My teacher was my kids for calling me out on my bullshit.

My teacher was John for pushing me to quit. Thanks for breaking the cycle with me for us and our family.

15. Authentically Free

My teacher was money for chasing and wanting more and not being happy with what I already had.

My teacher was being my body for starting to hurt, palpate, lose sleep, and have digestive problems.

My teacher was my drunk-ass friends. Seeing you with my sober eyes now is a whole other vibe. I don't want to be that person with you anymore. I'm still here for you but I can't be how I was in our previous relationship.

My teacher was myself. I'm in there, I'm rising out of the bullshit, I'm transforming into the woman I was meant to be. I can be a voice for a generation of women, my soul sisters – my '90s girls and our next generation.

It's fucking hard to go through all the shit layer by layer. Look at all the disgusting shit I have been through in my life.

I can honestly say that after quitting drinking more times than I can count, it was seriously just time for me to do it. There really is infinite wisdom in all of us and when it hits you, it's like a fucking brick wall and you just "know" this is it.

See, alcohol is tricky, it's like a sneaky little elf. It starts out innocent, sweet and fun then it turns into this soul sucking monster that convinces you there is something wrong with you that you are crazy or fucked up or an alcoholic. If you have experienced any of those thoughts or emotions don't beat yourself up for it. It wasn't you. He's a trickster, a thief, a liar. Alco elf did exactly what he intended to do.

I won, though, before it was too late.

I have attached myself to the term "Authentically Free." If you Google it, it just sort of talks about authenticity and being authentically "me."

What does "*authentic*" actually mean? It may be a little bit tricky to describe but it's actually very simple.

As per dictionary.com authentic is an adjective meaning "not false or copied; genuine; real:"

Miriam-Webster says, "True to one's own personality, spirit, or character."

Wow! Now how simple was that?

Super simple but we can break it down just one more slice.

Not false. Okay, so what's real? My definition would be... Not to be altered by any substance, not to put out a fake presence of who you are, to speak the truth, to honour your word, not trying to be someone that you are not. I can assure you that alcohol definitely makes you someone that you are not.

Now what does *"free"* mean? As per dictionary.com free is an adjective meaning, "enjoying personal rights or liberty as a person: independent: unrestricted." Miriam-webster says, "having liberty, not being interfered with or acted on by others, not subject to usual rules, obligations or restrictions." Dayuuummm that HITS!

So I'm looking to be unrestricted, independent, enjoying my personal rights and freedoms minus alcohol. Right?

While writing this, I feel that my soul is surfacing. My writing is cathartic in letting all of the bull shit go. This book is going to help hold and keep me accountable to my commitment to myself and my beautiful children.

Authentically free to me also means, stripping down. Not like we did to Christina Aguilera's *"Dirty"* at the club, but removing all of the layers that are covering our souls, our hearts. Being real and open. Allowing ourselves to breathe and know it's okay. We always hear about forgiveness and that it sets us free. Forgiveness to our mothers who abandoned us, forgiveness to those who have cheated on us, forgiveness to our bullies who fucked our entire existence in school, forgiveness towards our molesters, forgiveness towards anyone who has wronged us.

Forgiveness to flow through us, naturally without effort – to know in your being that it really wasn't about you – it was about them.

Speaking of you, it's your turn. Please forgive yourself. Make amends. The negative self talk needs to cease to exist. You are PERFECT just the way you are!

I promise!

15. Authentically Free

Apologize to yourself, write yourself a letter and honour yourself. Write that fucking letter. Let the booze know that you are pissed at it for making you do what you did, for saying what you said, for stealing what you stole, for fucking who you shouldn't have, for lying when you shouldn't have, for spending the money you shouldn't have, for giving you the worst hangovers, for making you do drugs.

Let it know everything that you are feeling.

Honour that you were influenced by sources outside of your immediate control. Forgive the alcohol. It was only doing what it was intending to do. It won – but only temporarily. It's your turn to win now.

Thank the booze. Thank it for the fun, for the good times, for the sexy boys (or girls) you kissed. Thank it for the lessons learned. Thank it for the awakenings, thank it for being in your life to remind you who you don't want to be, thank it for showing you the people that you don't want to surround yourself with.

Forgiveness is fucking hard! Trust me, I know! The mental chatter in our minds about having to forgive and accept. You don't have to do it face to face or even tell the person about it. You are doing this for you! I am forever grateful for the lessons learned. I am grateful for everything that has brought me to this place. I can own my story now. I can use my experiences to help others. I can be authentically free and that is the greatest gift of all.

So, my new friends, it's time to say goodbye to the past and hello to a brighter, authentic and free future. I'll raise my adulting trophy up high with you, as we cheers to living our best lives, free from the bondage of alcohol and living our truth. I much rather raise my figurative trophy high in the sky than cheers to a night I wish to forget.

That is true freedom, that is authenticity and that my dear soul sisters is a gift that we didn't know we needed, but have been searching for all of our lives. Us '90s girls have been through the ringer. I'm grateful to know that I have had all of the correct pieces all along. My pieces were just silenced.

The American Psychological Association dictionary states forgiveness as: "willfully putting aside feelings of resentment toward an individual who has committed a wrong, been unfair or hurtful, or otherwise harmed one in some way. Forgiveness is not equated with reconciliation or excusing another, and it is not merely accepting what happened or ceasing to be angry. Rather, it involves a voluntary transformation of one's feelings, attitudes, and behavior toward the individual, so that one is no longer dominated by resentment and can express compassion, generosity, or the like toward the individual. Forgiveness is sometimes considered an important process in psychotherapy or counseling."

I encourage you to read that again. I'm sure that all of the instances in your life that bring you hate and anger quite possibly may be some of the reasons you drink. There's a whole list of reasons to drink: my dad who was my best friend is gone, I had a shitty day at work, I didn't land the contract I wanted at work, I'm cooking, I'm not cooking, I'm relaxing, I'm so stressed out.

What about the reasons NOT to drink? There's a myriad of those too. Your kids, your job, your husband (or wife), so you don't drink and drive, so you don't spend a ridiculous amount of money, so you aren't depressed/anxious/overtired, for your physical health but most importantly for YOU – your authentic you, the real you who has hopes and dreams and aspirations. The YOU who knows all the shit that you have been through in your life. Taking charge of what's yours and what you can control, your life! You are making it. Do you know how I know? Because you are still here and for that I am grateful! Just think, dream a bit with me here for a minute. Just think of your wildest wishes, hopes and aspirations. Think about all of the new babies being born in the world, the beautiful sunsets, vacations, the scrapbooking that you keep putting off, the course you want to take and actually finish, the business you

15. Authentically Free

want to start, the money you want to make. You can literally do ANYTHING you want to if you can think it, have a burning desire to achieve it, and take action every single day to do something about it, it's yours!

You may have heard of the great philosopher Napoleon Hill. He is incredibly famous for his book, *Think And Grow Rich*.

He writes, *"Anything the human mind can believe, the human mind can achieve.* That is the Supreme Secret…. This is the secret known in bygone times; this is the secret which governs present-day accomplishment; this is the secret which will follow man to the stars. This is the secret of the ages."

Hill also has a list of 31 reasons that people fail in life. Here is reason 31:

Intemperance

"The most damaging forms of intemperance are connected with eating, strong drink, and sexual activities. Over-indulgence in any of these is fatal to success."

Intemperance as defined by vocabulary.com states that to be "Intemperate is a combination of the prefix in – meaning "not" and the Latin *temperantia* meaning "moderation." When you are intemperate, you are not doing things in moderation; you lack self-control. It's often a word used when describing the tendency someone has to indulge excessively in liquor."

To put the bottle down, knowing that I can truly have anything in my mind that I desire? Sign me up, baby! At least let me give it a solid effort. I mean what's the worst that can happen? I just MAY achieve greatness?

For the first time in my life I don't even have the temptation, so I have nothing to give into. I get to start every day with a clean slate – free from alcohol, free from the chaos it brings, free from the pain it was causing my kids. I can finally say with 100% certainty that I feel great in my own skin and that I'm free, truly authentically free.

Living authentically free is about embracing a lifestyle that aligns with your true self, values, and aspirations without the use of substances. It involves making conscious choices that contribute to your overall well-being, happiness, and personal growth. I encourage you to take a moment to read through these one by one, and repeat if needed as these ideas will help you on your journey as you hold your own heart.

1. Self-Reflection and Awareness

What motivates you? Maybe you can't answer that right now. You don't have any motivation. If you are still drinking then I'm not surprised that you don't have any motivation. I am, though, willing to bet that you DID have motivation when you were younger. Go back to that place. What did you want to be when you grew up? What did you like learning about? Do you have kids? Do they motivate you? I bet you love your kids without a shadow of a doubt. I get you. It wasn't solely my children who made me put the bottle down. Them alone wasn't enough. That's hard to admit. They were, however, a part of the process and my motivation for why I needed to. I needed to be motivated by many things, not just one. What motivates you and how is alcohol helping you stay motivated? Find your strengths, weaknesses, and passions. Write them down. These will help to guide your life choices.

2. Embracing Emotions

People drink for two reasons. They drink either to feel "something" or to feel nothing. I was in the "something" category. Being pushed into maturity unintentionally by my mothers emotional absence and disease, led me to suppressing my childhood and my inner child's feelings. That stuck with me and I became a hard ass. Emotionless throughout my life and relationships. I would drink to feel music, love, to feel inspired. To feel something, anything. Not drinking isn't the only thing that will change your life. On its own, quitting drinking didn't make me a better mom or human. It was the learning I did and continue to do. The therapy I'm going to, the positive actions and reactions around my family, the community that I'm building. I no longer hang out with people that drink. Jim Rohn once said, "You are the average of the five people you spend the most time with." Makes perfect sense to me. If you surround yourselves with drunks you will become one. Could you imagine being wasted in a room with Oprah, Albert Einstein, Tony Robbins, Wayne Dyer and Mother Teresa? I don't believe it would ever happen! Chances are if they were all in a room together you definitely wouldn't go for the bottle. Choose your five people wisely. They have the potential to change your life.

It's okay to allow yourself to experience a range of emotions without the need to numb or suppress them. We can try as hard as possible, but all suppressed emotions will show up down the road. It could be five years or it could be 30 years. They show up in many shapes and forms such as anger, solitude, ocd, resentment, etc… Adhering to healthy coping mechanisms to navigate challenging feelings and situations is a superpower that will enable you to be your best self.

3. Building Authentic Connections

It's imperative that we cultivate genuine relationships based on shared interests, values, and mutual respect. Connecting with others on a deeper level, fostering meaningful relationships without the influence of alcohol.

If you have a roommate that just wants to party and is wasted all the time while you just want a quiet place to call home then the harsh reality is you need a new roommate! Moving through sobriety is a lot easier when you change your environment. I can promise you that if I wasn't locked in a hotel room for four days at the beginning of all this I wouldn't be where I am today. Literally changing my physical environment was instrumental in launching my journey of sobriety.

4. Exploring Personal Passions

I had really suppressed my passion for writing/journaling over the past 10 years. I wrote a little bit but it was never enough to fulfill me like it used to. Putting the bottle down launched the writing of this book. I got back to what I was passionate about. This book has me connecting with new and old friends who are now sober. This book makes me feel that I have a sense of purpose aside from only being a mother, that I am fulfilling my own dharma. This book is bringing me back to when I was happy as a coach and helping people. I'm pursuing personal and professional goals with a clear and focused mindset. Who knows where this book is going to go or who's hands it will end up in but I remain hopeful that it lands in the hands of someone who needs and will benefit from it.

5. Mindful Living

It's so hard to be mindful in our lives, when we poison our soul. Practice mindfulness and present living, appreciating each moment without the fog of substances. I will keep it short here because I really get into what it means to live with a mindful purpose in a later chapter called "Mindful Path To Recovery" where we learn to engage in activities with full awareness, fostering a deeper connection to our experiences and our true self.

6. Cultivating a Healthy Lifestyle

Prioritizing your physical health through regular exercise, balanced nutrition, and adequate sleep is a GAME CHANGER! It's incredible how when we eliminate the poisons in our life, we become witness to some pretty incredible positive miracles.

Now that I'm sleeping properly I don't need to have a nap to deal with my life or children. I don't detest anymore even just simple chores like doing the laundry! I'm not overloading my organs with an excess of liquid carbs, then carb filled take out food until I have a lump of food in my body before I pass out and expect my body to process it while I'm sleeping. When you can kick one bad habit like drinking, it's automatic that you just naturally start kicking other habits because you can see and feel the benefits almost instantly. If you can curb one addiction you can curb many, sometimes without even being cognisant about it. Another byproduct of sobriety.

7. Authentic Self-Expression

This could take some work! Especially if your self expression has been attached to alcohol. You are so fun and exciting, the life of the party and so likeable. Until you are not. Part of the reason you are reading this book. Expressing your thoughts, opinions, and creativity without inhibition. That's super easy to do when we are drinking. Does that usually end up in anger? It certainly did for me. I rarely went to bed happy after a night of drinking.

Who are you? How do you embrace your unique identity and celebrate your individuality without alcohol? Ask your friends… Your REAL friends. Not your drinking buddies. Who do they think you are when you are sober? That's the real you. THOSE are the attributes you need to work on and grow. Are you a writer? An artist? Do you love animals? Do you like to help people? How can you do more of that? That's how you will fill your soul and express your true self.

8. Setting Boundaries

Establishing and maintaining healthy boundaries in relationships is vitally important to respecting your own needs and recovery.

You absolutely have the right to say "no" to situations or people that compromise your authenticity, sobriety or well-being. People in your life are not on the same path or journey as you. You know how I know this? Well, because they aren't you! It's pretty simple. If your friends want to go out partying, let them! If they want to be upset with you for not attending an event where alcohol is going to be served, let them! You see where I'm going here? Let them do whatever they want but that means you have to let yourself do what you want that enables you to move forward in a healthy trajectory while prioritizing your sobriety. No is a complete sentence.

You may lose some people along the way. They may not see a benefit to your friendship anymore and they may slip out the back door. Let them! Some of your Facebook "friends" might stop liking your posts. Let them!

It's time to stop living your life on other people's terms.

9. Ongoing Personal Growth

Embracing a mindset of continual self-improvement and growth is vital to your sobriety and longevity. What does this look like for you? Go back to number one... Self-Reflection and Awareness, and really do an assessment on your life and goals.

A tree can only grow from its own roots. Yes, anyone can water it. They can "water" it with water, Kool-aid, pop or in our case alcohol. The latter three would certainly impact its growth or hinder it all together with the right amounts. But its roots (soul) and just plain ol' water are what will keep it stable and continue to reach for its goal, the sun.

Think of your soul as the roots. The tree intuitively knows where it's going. Up...

Your soul wants the best for you! It wants to succeed, it wants to grow and be nourished with positivity and love.

We can learn from our experiences within our journey through drinking and substance abuse. Through these experiences, challenges, and setbacks, we must use them as opportunities for education and development.

Reach For The Sun!

10. Living in Alignment with Values

Can you even identify what your values are? If you asked me a few years ago what my values were I couldn't even tell you. I would give you the expected answers of "I value my friends and family." That's probably it. I have since learned to identify and uphold personal values that guide my decisions and actions.

For example, I value my sobriety because it aligns with the life that I want to live and enables me to achieve my goals.

I value my assertiveness. This shows strength and confidence while staying respectful to myself and others. I believe in speaking up for what I believe is right and to be confident in my decisions without being influenced negatively by others opinions.

Values are really things that you believe are important for the way you live your life and work such as... courage, dependability, family traditions and beliefs as well as generosity and gratitude.

I'm constantly working on ensuring that my lifestyle choices align with my principles and beliefs= my values.

11. Authenticity in Social Settings

If you can live within your values that you have set out for yourself, this can enable you the strength to navigate social situations confidently without the reliance of substances for social interactions. If you feel that you are unable to attend an event without the use of substances I would suggest re-evaluating your events, your friends and your situations. You want to be building connections based on genuine interactions, shared interests, and positive energy. It starts with you and your values. Your values will be a roadmap on how to navigate throughout your life. When faced with challenges, ask yourself... Do these people, events or situations line up with my values? If yes, then you are heading in the right direction, if no then you know what you need to do.

Your friends, co-workers and family should love you regardless of whether you are drinking or not. If they chose to drink, that's up to them although we both know what the end of the night is going to look like for them, so believe me when I say you are making the right decision to stay home or to go and have a good time without drinking alcohol. You can do this! Change is hard especially when you are confronted with the fact that people knew you a certain way. Your sober way though, is new and improved which is 100% more likeable. You, 2.0!

12. Celebrating Achievements

Each day in sobriety is a huge day. Even if you have "only" been sober for a day... That's a HUGE win! That's a whole 24 hours where poison didn't enter your body. That's 1440 minutes or 86400 seconds! Holy shit.... What a big number. Acknowledge and celebrate milestones and accomplishments in your discovery to living authentically free. Your small wins are bigger than you think.

Getting and staying sober requires strength and resilience that you may not have known you needed or had. Yes, you do have it in you, yes, it's going to be a lot of fucking work... Every day and probably for the rest of your life. There have been millions of people before you and there will be millions of people after you who have chosen or will choose to get sober... Now that's a statistic you want to be a part of. Never quit quitting! One day you will have learned your lesson and you will no longer need the teacher because you *Woke Up One Day & Changed Your F★cking Mind!*

It's impossible to live authentically, (which is what we all want to be loved for, really) while being drunk. They just don't go together, like fire and gasoline. Living authentically while being sober is about embracing a life that feels true to who you are, allowing you to thrive and experience fulfillment on your own terms. It's a journey of self-discovery, self-acceptance, and intentional living.

Never quit quitting!

CHAPTER 16

The How, Who, What, Where, but MOST importantly HOW?

Now I know that you know that you NEED to quit drinking. I knew for years that I needed to, too. For some reason I just couldn't stop – aside from the whole alcohol being a poison and trapping me a bit. I just kept going back.

I think for me, actually… I know for me near the end that it was just a habit more than anything really. The habit of getting home from work and grabbing the wine, the habit of cooking and grabbing the wine, the nightly habit of sitting on the porch and drinking wine, the habit of folding laundry and drinking wine, the habit of cleaning and drinking wine, the habit of gardening and drinking wine (or having a Corona), the habit of just going to the pub after work, drinking vodka crans, the habit of drinking with the neighbors.

I really didn't need booze to do any of those things. Part and parcel, drinking would give me a temporary energy boost to get those things done. It's not like I would drop dead without the booze from lack of energy. No one forced me to go to the liquor store. I didn't get the shakes and NEED the booze. *Brain Wow* moment – it was literally just a habit… Does this sound familiar?

We get conditioned to develop our habits. Our childhood conditioning, our trauma response conditioning, our societal conditioning. But is there ALWAYS something to blame for conditioning? I'm no psychologist, psychiatrist or therapist but maybe in some cases we just sort of start the new patterns in a family, in a generation.

I have been to therapy in my life a lot! More specifically over the past couple of years I kept saying, "when will I fully process my childhood" and "I've processed my molestation. I'm seriously done talking about it."

Most of me wants to believe that I drank because it was habitual, it was routine. That I had complete control over it when I WANTED to, but I never wanted to. It was fun! What I didn't have control over was being able to stop after I started, so that's where the addiction came in. I'm throwing out a new term here if it doesn't already exist but I'm going with "Habitually Addicted To Alcohol."

Once I started drinking, Alco Elf started working up his wizardry and a glass of wine turned into two bottles, into 2 am, into $10,000k in the hole, into a fucking shit show.

If my hangovers were really bad, I would skip a day, no problem. Well, actually all the problems because I physically couldn't move. On a good hangover day (if that's even a thing) for the most part, I would hangover my day away functioning "normally" then start cooking and get into the wine to feel MY "normal", which was energetic, chatty, excited, etc.

Maybe you didn't have parents who were alcoholics so you don't have that to blame?

Maybe you didn't experience any childhood trauma?

Maybe you had an amazing childhood full of love, laughter and family?

Maybe you took your first drink 5, 10 years ago, and now you have a problem because you just got into the habit of it. Weddings=drinking, birthdays=drinking, friends over=drinking, out for a meal=drinking.

Is it okay not to blame our past for our current conditioning or conditions?

I think it totally is (now again I'm no trained professional), but I keep going back to the molestation and my emotionally absent mother... Like seriously? Say I kept drinking until I was

16. The How, Who, What, Where, but MOST importantly HOW?

70. I'm going to say it was because I was suppressing feelings from my childhood. I'm sorry but I call bullshit. Especially because of all the work I have done to heal.

I got into the daily habit, then the addiction would kick in and I couldn't stop until the bottle was gone (it certainly wasn't my childhood trauma making me drink). Do you see where I'm coming from here? Maybe not and you don't agree. That's fine. I'm just shedding light on where I'm at.

I feel the same about cocaine. There were days in a row where I'd be drinking and then get into the cocaine on night one, then night two, then three and four.... It was a short-lived habit for the benders I was on but during the bender after that first line the addiction kicks in and I just wanted more. I couldn't stop! I was habitually addicted or addicted to my habit.

Maybe you have some apprehensions about quitting? Are you thinking about what your life is going to look like? For the most part a LOT of us have the same routines (or habits) of events that we do every day, ie scenario 1: Get up at 6, go pee, shower, get dressed, go to work, pick up kids, start supper, watch TV, get ready for bed then do it all again. Insert your booze consumption anywhere in there – that's fine...

Now let's look at it this way, scenario 2: Get up at 6, shower, get dressed, then go pee, go to work, start supper then pick up kids, get ready for bed, then watch TV.

Super weird to change up your habits like that, right? Of course, it is! You have probably been living scenario 1 for forever (maybe a different pattern of events but you rarely or never switch to scenario 2).

For me getting out of the ordinary, getting out of my house, getting away from my kitchen (cooking was a trigger for me). Going on the work trip and being in a hotel for a month is what did it for me. I had to completely change my surroundings so that I could break the HABIT.

Now am I saying you have to run away and live in a hotel for a month? No but, have you ever thought about it? Did it ever cross your mind that "If I could just be by myself for a little bit and get away from the craziness of my day to day life I could get a grip of this stupid thing?"

Well, maybe I am, maybe I'm not saying run away for a month? If it's an option for you to just go away and leave the chaos of your life to just be alone and really do the dirty work to break yourself free, then go fucking do it! If it's time for rehab then go fucking do it! People aren't going to judge you negatively for fixing your life and if they do, you need new people. Sobriety requires a lot of restructuring of your surroundings. You have to change things in your life if you want or expect your life to change.

Hang out by yourself, detox, roll around like a lifeless depressed piece of shit listening to *Friends* reruns or audiobooks on sobriety and changing your life and slowly emerge as you finally decide to have a shower on day 4. That first shower washes away a layer of guilt and shame. You still have a ton of work to do but it's been 4 days. If you can do 4, then you can do 8. If you can do 8, then you can do 16.

Start going for walks. Go into some shops you have never been to, journal or read in a park, go to a bookstore, get a sobriety tattoo (I did), do SOMETHING, anything but drink. Start building your new life! Get excited about being sober the same way you got excited about being drunk… Let's focus our attention on what's helpful in fulfilling our goals, reaching our full potential while maintaining our values.

Please note* *If you are so far into your addiction and have developed a dependance for substances I do NOT recommend this route. Please see your doctor for an appropriate course of action.*

If you do make the decision to get help at a treatment facility or check in to a hotel, your family will be okay. I really doubt your husband/boyfriend/wife would leave you for taking care of your physical, mental and emotional well-being. With that said, if you do leave please let your family know what you are doing and let them know where you are at and that you are okay.

16. The How, Who, What, Where, but MOST importantly HOW?

I can promise you (from experience) that your family will NOT be okay if you continue down the path of self destruction. It's funny… They call it "self-destruction" but in actuality alcohol has the amazing power to destroy literally everyone and everything it's around, not just self.

If it is not an option for you to run away for a few – that's okay too. You aren't stuck. I promise. Either way you chose to tackle this beast – at home in your current surroundings or you dip out for a little while you can do it. It's either going to be hard work now or harder work later on but still work that needs to get done. Let's stop bringing today's shit into tomorrow.

"Okay… So I've decided to get sober. I've sort of got a game plan but I still have questions."

Well, I'm here to help.

Hence the title of this chapter. I'm going to try and help you talk through anything and everything that may be coming up for you. Let's unpack this shit right now. Once we get to the end, I want you to look in the mirror and see what excuse you can come up with for why you will "quit on Monday" and not today.

I encourage you to get a notebook or your journal, or just a sheet of paper to write these questions down on. Do it now and do it again in 6 months and see how your answer will change. I promise you will be pleasantly surprised.

This is a very comprehensive list of questions to navigate through as you are on your journey through sobriety or are contemplating living authentically free. Don't rush through them. Answer them honestly.

These questions are here for you to take the time for you to reflect on you, your past, your present and the best that is yet to come – your future. Living sober is a whole new vibe. Change CAN be scary but it doesn't always have to be. I said it before and I'll say it again… There have been millions of people before you, millions of people going through it now and millions of people after you who have faced the decision and who will face the decision to kick the booze.

Let's *Wake You Up & Change Your Fucking Mind*!

Take a deep breath, focus on you – exhale, relax…

Here we go!

HOW?

Quitting drinking is a significant decision that can bring about various challenges and reflections. Asking yourself certain questions can help you navigate this process and gain insights into your motivations, feelings, and goals. Here are some "how" questions you might want to add to your arsenal that will help to enable you to finally *Wake Up One Day & Change Your F*cking Mind*:

1. How will I cope with stress and difficult emotions without relying on alcohol?
2. How can I build a support system to help me stay accountable during this process?
3. How will I handle social situations where alcohol is present?
4. How can I create a healthier daily routine that doesn't involve drinking?
5. How will I manage potential triggers that may tempt me to drink?
6. How can I educate myself about the physical and mental benefits of sobriety?
7. How will I celebrate achievements and milestones without turning to alcohol?
8. How can I replace the time and energy spent on drinking with positive and fulfilling activities?
9. How will I communicate my decision to quit drinking to friends and family?
10. How can I establish new habits and hobbies that support a sober lifestyle?

11. How will I address any underlying issues or reasons that led to excessive drinking?
12. How can I stay motivated and focused on my goal during challenging times?
13. How will I navigate the potential social pressures or expectations related to drinking?
14. How can I learn from past experiences with alcohol and use them to propel my commitment to sobriety?
15. How will I handle setbacks or relapses with a positive and constructive mindset?
16. How can I find alternative ways to relax and unwind without turning to alcohol?
17. How will I prioritize self-care and mental health during this transition?
18. How can I cultivate a sense of purpose and fulfillment in my life without relying on alcohol?
19. How will I deal with cravings and temptations in a healthy and proactive manner?
20. How can I continually reassess and adjust my strategies for maintaining a sober lifestyle?

Holy shit right? Did I read your mind? Have you been contemplating some, if not all of these scenarios? There's a lot there to think about. Now did you one word answer those questions? If you did go back. You missed the memo. These questions as exercises are designed to make you go somewhere uncomfortable, to dig and really start figuring shit out. Learning to build skills and values for the authentic you that is in there. These are tools for your toolbox to constantly reflect on.

WHO

People need people. There's definitely no refuting that. We often get stuck with the people in our lives and convince ourselves that we don't have the choice of who is present in our lives. For some reason we forget that we have the right to choose how people treat us, by setting our own personal boundaries and deciding for a FACT what behaviour, actions and words will be tolerated or welcomed in our lives by others.

Certainly, understanding the social aspects and interpersonal dynamics related to quitting drinking is crucial. Here are some "who" questions you need to consider asking yourself in order to prioritize your sobriety.

1. Who are the supportive individuals in my life who can help me on this journey?
2. Who are the people I need to communicate my decision to quit drinking, and how will I approach these conversations?
3. Who can be my accountability partner or support system during challenging times?
4. Who are the friends or acquaintances who may influence me negatively in terms of drinking, and how will I manage those relationships?
5. Who are the positive role models or individuals who have successfully quit drinking that I can learn from?
6. Who can I engage with in activities that don't involve alcohol, fostering a healthier social life?
7. Who in my social circle understands the importance of my decision and will respect it?
8. Who might be open to joining me in adopting a healthier lifestyle or participating in alcohol-free events?
9. Who are the professionals or support groups that I can turn to for guidance and assistance?
10. Who are the people I can lean on for emotional support when dealing with the challenges of quitting drinking?
11. Who will be part of my new, sober social network?
12. Who are the individuals I need to establish boundaries with regarding alcohol-related activities?

13. Who are the family members or close friends who may need education about the significance of my decision?
14. Who can I turn to for encouragement and positive reinforcement when I achieve milestones in my sobriety?
15. Who are the people I can engage with in activities that align with my new, alcohol-free lifestyle?
16. Who are the potential triggers or stressors in my life, and how will I manage interactions with them without turning to alcohol?
17. Who can provide guidance on rebuilding relationships that may have been strained due to past drinking behavior?
18. Who are the professionals or experts I can consult for advice on mental health and coping strategies during this transition?
19. Who can help me identify and address any underlying issues contributing to my drinking habits?
20. Who are the individuals I can turn to for understanding and empathy if I face judgment or skepticism about my decision to quit drinking? Maybe one or more of these people are people you need to extend an apology to in order to forgive yourself and to attempt to heal who you have hurt.

Asking yourself these "who" questions can help you build a supportive network and navigate the social aspects of your journey through sobriety. This may mean that some people that have been in your life are not a suitable fit to continue being in your life and that is okay.

I was one of those people for someone who was sober from alcohol and cocaine. I was a shitty friend. I did it around her and actually ended up convincing her to drink. It wasn't long until she kicked me to the curb. Rightfully so.

I did reach out to her where I attempted to make amends and to apologize for my actions. At the time of this writing she hasn't read the message.

Maybe someday, somehow she will see this. It will be okay if she doesn't respond but I would like her to know that I am truly sorry.

If you need some inspiration to write your I'm sorry note… Here's mine.

> Hey Kim,
>
> I just wanted to apologize to you for bringing you around the chaos that surrounded me with my alcohol abuse and drug use – especially when you got sober. It was selfish and not supportive. You were always a good friend to me and I broke your trust. So for that I'm truly sorry. You look amazing. I'm proud of you for staying strong and true to yourself! I too am sober now and happier than ever. It only took 20+ years. Still with John and have 2 more kids. I miss you and hope you are still doing amazing and crushing life!
>
> Love, Challaine

Simple, direct, apologetic and honest. It's now up to her to do what she wants with it. I'm not going to beg for her friendship but at least I know I have taken the steps needed in order to begin to repair, if possible.

WHAT

Certainly, asking yourself "what" questions can help you clarify your goals, identify strategies, and focus on specific aspects of your journey to quit drinking. Here are some "what" to consider when choosing sobriety:

1. What are my primary motivations for quitting drinking?
2. What specific challenges do I anticipate encountering, and how can I prepare for them?

3. What changes do I need to make in my daily routine to support a sober lifestyle?
4. What strategies will I employ to cope with stress and difficult emotions without turning to alcohol?
5. What are the potential triggers for my drinking, and how can I avoid or manage them?
6. What new habits or hobbies can I adopt to replace the time and energy spent on drinking?
7. What resources, such as books, articles, or support groups, can I utilize to educate myself about sobriety?
8. What positive affirmations or mantras can I incorporate into my daily routine to stay motivated?
9. What milestones or achievements will I celebrate as I progress in my journey to quit drinking?
10. What alternative beverages or activities will I explore to fill the void left by alcohol?
11. What kind of support do I need from friends, family, or professionals, and how can I communicate this effectively?
12. What is my plan for handling social situations where alcohol is present?
13. What role will exercise and physical activity play in supporting my overall well-being during this transition?
14. What coping mechanisms or relaxation techniques will I employ when facing cravings or temptations?
15. What steps can I take to repair relationships that may have been affected by my drinking habits?
16. What healthy boundaries do I need to establish with friends or acquaintances who still drink?
17. What steps can I take to address any underlying issues contributing to my drinking behavior?
18. What kind of self-reflection practices will I incorporate into my routine to stay mindful of my progress?

19. What will be my response if I encounter setbacks or relapses along the way?
20. What long-term goals do I have for my physical and mental well-being after quitting drinking?

These "what" questions can guide you in defining your objectives, developing a plan, and maintaining focus on your path to sobriety.

WHERE

You have the choice to choose where you put your body. Like actually. If putting yourself in situations that disables your sobriety journey then you need to make different choices, because your physical and mental health depends on it!

Asking yourself "where" questions can help you consider the environmental and situational aspects of your journey to quit drinking. Here are some "where" questions you might find useful:

1. Where are the locations or environments that trigger my desire to drink, and how can I minimize my exposure to them?
2. Where will I find support groups or meetings to connect with others who are also on a journey to quit drinking?
3. Where can I discover alcohol-free social events or activities to participate in?
4. Where will I go when I need a safe and supportive space during challenging times in my sobriety?
5. Where can I find resources, such as books or online materials, that provide information and guidance on quitting drinking?
6. Where will I create my sober sanctuary or space for self-reflection and mindfulness?

16. THE HOW, WHO, WHAT, WHERE, BUT MOST IMPORTANTLY HOW?

7. Where are the places where I can engage in new hobbies or activities that don't involve alcohol?
8. Where can I locate professionals or counselors who specialize in addiction and can provide additional support?
9. Where will I establish boundaries with friends or acquaintances who continue to drink?
10. Where are the venues or events that promote a healthier, alcohol-free lifestyle?
11. Where can I explore alternative beverages or non-alcoholic options that I enjoy?
12. Where are the supportive friends or family members I can turn to during moments of temptation or struggle?
13. Where will I go for physical activities or exercise to improve my overall well-being during this transition?
14. Where can I find alcohol-free social networks or online communities for additional support and advice?
15. Where will I celebrate milestones and achievements in my journey to quit drinking?
16. Where are the places or situations where I feel most vulnerable to relapse, and how can I navigate them effectively?
17. Where can I establish new connections with individuals who support and understand my decision to quit drinking?
18. Where will I seek professional help if I encounter challenges that I cannot overcome on my own?
19. Where can I engage in self-reflection practices or mindfulness activities to stay connected to my sobriety goals?
20. Where do I envision myself in the future, free from the influence of alcohol, and how will I work towards that vision?

These "where" questions can help you identify and shape your physical and social environments to support your commitment to quitting drinking.

WHY

This section you may find yourself asking more often than the others. Asking yourself "why" questions is crucial for understanding your motivations, reinforcing your commitment, and gaining insight into the reasons behind your decision to quit drinking. Here are some "why" questions to consider when you are faced with the choice of sobriety or alcoholism:

1. Why do I want to quit drinking in the first place?
2. Why is sobriety important to my overall well-being and happiness?
3. Why have past attempts to quit drinking not been successful, and what can I learn from those experiences?
4. Why do I believe quitting drinking will positively impact my relationships with others?
5. Why do I want to break free from the cycle of dependence on alcohol?
6. Why is it essential for me to prioritize my physical and mental health at this point in my life?
7. Why do I think sobriety will contribute to my personal growth and self-improvement?
8. Why do I want to eliminate alcohol as a coping mechanism for stress or difficult emotions?
9. Why do I believe quitting drinking will lead to a more fulfilling and purposeful life?
10. Why is it important for me to be a positive influence on those around me, especially friends and family?
11. Why do I want to regain control over my actions and decisions without the influence of alcohol?

12. Why is it crucial for me to address any underlying issues or traumas that may contribute to my drinking habits?
13. Why do I value the idea of living authentically and true to myself without the crutch of alcohol?
14. Why is it essential to break free from the societal expectations or pressures related to drinking?
15. Why do I believe sobriety will enhance my mental clarity, focus, and overall cognitive function?
16. Why is it important for me to be a positive role model for others who may be struggling with similar challenges?
17. Why do I want to create a healthier and more sustainable lifestyle for myself?
18. Why do I believe sobriety will lead to more meaningful and genuine connections with others?
19. Why is it crucial for me to invest in my long-term physical and mental well-being?
20. Why do I want to prove to myself that I have the strength and resilience to overcome the challenges of quitting drinking?

Reflecting on these "why" questions can help you solidify your motivations and provide a strong foundation for your journey through sobriety. This isn't just a one time deal. Asking yourself these questions regularly can amplify your decisions to keep moving through your sobriety.

I told you I had a comprehensive list for you. Those were good, weren't they? How did it feel to think about those ideas? You had to put yourself first in a lot of those scenarios. Just like you put yourself first with your drinking, all we're doing here is changing direction and putting yourself first in order for you to get healthy, feel energetic, feel alive and live life to the fullest in your day to day.

Feel free to go back to this list and use it as part of your affirmations as you go throughout your day.

Chances are people are going to ask you about why you have chosen or are choosing sobriety. It's going to feel awkward and you are definitely going to get asked one or more of the following…

"Why did you quit drinking"?

"Are you an alcoholic? Is that why you quit"?

"How much were you drinking"?

Even though it really doesn't matter to anyone else that you decided to quit drinking, the perfect answer that I have found is, *I Just Woke Up One Day & Changed My F*cking Mind.*

Feel free to use that for yourself if you like. I find it pretty empowering for me when I say it.

As complicated as it can be, it really is that simple. It may take hitting rock bottom once or several times for you to quit or you literally may have just had enough and your innate wisdom and intuition will lead you to quit.

For me I hit rock bottom many times. But it was never enough. The cops being at my house multiple times throughout several relationships, physically assaulting my ex, going to jail, abusing drugs, all the hangovers, vomit, suicidal thoughts and excessive gambling, etc. Some may call all of those instances rock bottom. To me it was just "another day at the office" I suppose. None of those were really out of the ordinary, it was all just par for the course.

Looking back, in the moment I would always have an excuse of why all that negative shit was happening. None of those instances were MY fault, even though I was involved in every single one. Uh-huh! The lies we tell ourselves.

Weird how our minds make us so right all the time when we are drinking. I mean seriously. It was MY fault that I assaulted my ex (regardless of what he said/did). It was MY fault that the cops showed up to my house on more than one occasion. I was involved in every situation, so how could I blame someone else? Oh, the naivety.

16. THE HOW, WHO, WHAT, WHERE, BUT MOST IMPORTANTLY HOW?

The Most Important HOW – How Do You Quit?

I don't want to be a Debbie downer. I don't. If I had the answer for you then we would all be able to get sober no problem and "battling" alcohol abuse or addiction wouldn't be a thing and I wouldn't be writing this book.

I wish I could take away all of the hurt and the pain that you and everyone is going through (maybe that's the mother in me) but I also know for some fucking reason you have to go through all the bullshit (maybe thats the mother in me too). Just like with my kids. When they get hurt, when they have a breakup, when anything affects them so bad that it hurts their heart. I wish I could take it from them but I know, like I had to, they just have to experience it. Like a right of passage or something into adulthood. I can only be there to offer support and be a sounding board for them.

I hope it doesn't take hitting rock bottom once (or 10 times like me) to quit.

I wish there was a quick fix to this problem. You're like me and we just want a quick fix. Hey! I know you.

It hurts and it's fucking hard. Just like a breakup with a partner you have to go "through" it. When I think of ending my relationship with alcohol. There's LOTS of moving pieces. If you're like me, it was a long relationship. It is a breakup. It was a part of you, your life, your routine. But just like you went through your break ups and ended up okay or even better than okay… You HAVE to go through the process of breaking up with alcohol my friend.

Through…

That's how.

CHAPTER 17

Quitting Cold Turkey VS Drinking Responsibly

What comes to mind when you hear the term "drink responsibly"? That short little phrase is at the end of every alcohol commercial on TV, you see it in restrooms at the bar or pub. But what does it actually mean to you?

For me, during my whole life as a habitually addictive drinker my mind never reached further than "drink responsibly" means "don't drink and drive."

Like seriously – that's it!

Holy fuck! Now that's pretty narrow-minded, eh? Possibly, but we only know what we are taught. When we are continually taught the same things over and over again, especially from a young age they become our truth or reality.

We have a nationwide program here in Canada called MADD, Mothers Against Drunk Driving. I remember their commercials in grade school about the dangers of drinking and driving. I remember the police coming to school and talking about drinking and driving. No one, and I mean NO ONE ever talked about the other consequences of drinking, like the social, physical, financial, and mental consequences of drinking alcohol. So it was kind of ingrained in us that alcohol was okay as long as we didn't drink and drive.

Still, as I continue to write this book I've been sober for 20 days and that's fucking awesome! Going from 2 bottles a night – every night to nothing cold turkey. For me I've always been an all or nothing kinda gal. Not "have a glass of wine with supper." There was no way I could have just one glass. For the sake of this conversation, though, quitting cold turkey was right for me. This is what I felt at the time. I wanted it done, over with, I had serious physical work to do. I couldn't wean myself off. I didn't want to wean myself off. Just get it done!

I have quit boozing cold turkey before and it has always worked for me, until I justified getting into it again and again. Quitting cold turkey is fine for the short term but if you don't do the work to actually quit then you are just quitting between drinks.

To save my own ass and the ass of you my beautiful reader, this cold turkey approach is however… NOT RECOMMENDED!

I did know the risks prior to quitting and decided to go against the grain.

Please read the following list as potential consequences from quitting drinking abruptly.

I know what you are probably thinking, "I'm damned if I do, I'm damned if I don't (quit drinking)"… Trust me, you will be more damned if you do continue a life of alcoholism.

So, here is my due diligence recommending that you don't quit cold turkey. Everyone's health is different, consumption/absorption rate is different, tolerance is different, etc.

Here are some reasons why quitting alcohol cold turkey may be problematic for you.

1. Withdrawal Symptoms
- Alcohol withdrawal symptoms can range from mild to severe, depending on the level of dependence. Abrupt cessation can lead to symptoms such as tremors, anxiety, nausea, insomnia, and, in severe cases, seizures.

    (for me – anxiety and insomnia)

2. Delirium Tremens (DTs)
- In some cases, sudden cessation of alcohol in individuals with a high level of dependence can lead to a severe and life-threatening condition called delirium tremens. DTs

symptoms may include hallucinations, severe confusion, and cardiovascular issues.

(I had very, very mild hallucinations of people/objects that weren't actually there, but they appeared in my periphery).

3. Medical Complications

- Quitting alcohol suddenly can lead to medical complications such as dehydration, electrolyte imbalances, and nutritional deficiencies, which may require medical intervention.

Severe dehydration for me. My pee would stink like a nursing home – surprise! Most people in nursing homes are dehydrated. I was definitely deprived of nutrients – as mentioned in my earlier chapter that the soul sucking poison also sucked major nutrients out of my body which led to just feeling like shit all the time. My reserves were empty. I'm still working on getting them back up with supplementation and eating properly.

4. Increased Risk of Relapse

- Abruptly stopping alcohol without proper support or a plan in place may increase the risk of relapse, as you may find it challenging managing withdrawal symptoms without assistance.

(So far so good – actually so far so EXCELLENT!)

5. Psychological Impact

- The sudden removal of alcohol can have a significant impact on someone's mental health, potentially leading to increased anxiety, depression, or irritability.

I went through a major depression when I quit but thankfully the severity of it only lasted about 4 days. Drinking was the only thing that would make the depression in my life go away. Knowing this would justify picking up the bottle again. I had to hermit in my bed, sulk, roll around and mope. Super shitty times, but hey! Look at me now.

I'm writing a fucking book!!! I wouldn't trade those four days for anything. I had to get through those days to have the clarity to be here and write my heart out to you today.

6. Safety Concerns
- For those with a severe dependence on alcohol, attempting to quit cold turkey without medical supervision can pose safety risks, especially if complications such as seizures or DTs occur or if you have previous medical conditions.

    (I never had a true physical dependence on alcohol. It was habitual for me. Some people do have the NEED for alcohol in order for them not to have severe withdrawal symptoms/complications).

7. Lack of Support
- Quitting alcohol without a support system or treatment plan may result in feelings of isolation, making it more difficult for you to cope with the challenges of sobriety.

    * I LOVE and thrive on alone time. Being by myself during the early days of my sobriety was optimal for me. Provided John was around as we were in a hotel room (still are 20 days later). He gave me the space I needed and wanted. I also created my own sober community. I have had a real fine balance of solitude and support from others which has helped me thrive.

8. Underlying Health Issues
- You may have underlying health conditions that can be exacerbated by abrupt alcohol cessation. Seeking professional guidance ensures a comprehensive understanding of your health status.

    (I don't have any underlying medical concerns).

9. Risk for Self-Medication
- Quitting alcohol cold turkey might lead some to self-medicate with other substances, potentially replacing one dependency with another.

    (I was advised to take my antidepressants. I took one and that was it)

Here's what you can to consider Instead of quitting cold turkey:

1. Consult a Healthcare Professional
- Before making any decisions about quitting alcohol, consult with a healthcare professional, such as a doctor or addiction specialist, to assess your individual situation and receive guidance on a suitable approach.

2. Medical Detox
- In cases of moderate to severe alcohol dependence, a supervised medical detoxification program may be recommended. This involves tapering off alcohol with medical oversight to manage withdrawal symptoms safely.

3. Treatment Programs
- Consider enrolling in a structured treatment program, such as an inpatient or outpatient rehabilitation facility, where you can receive support, counseling, and medical supervision during the recovery process.

4. Support Groups
- Joining support groups, such as Alcoholics Anonymous (AA), can provide valuable assistance and encouragement from individuals who have gone through similar experiences. There are a TON of social media pages surrounding sobriety. As I was rolling around in my own self-pity the first few days, all the scrolling happened. I joined so many sobriety pages and found so much motivation and inspiration of what I could do with my life,

what it would look like being sober and also who I didn't want to be.

5. Therapy and Counseling
- Engage in therapy or counseling to address the psychological aspects of alcohol dependence and develop coping strategies for maintaining sobriety.

(I talked with my therapist on and off about my drinking for over a year. My last session before I left for this work trip she gave me sort of like a road map sheet with about 20 rectangles on it. I was to write down some of my major life events. This was going to help us unpack some shit to see why I was at where I was at. Well, there's that all or nothing thing again. I didn't write anything on that paper. I started a book to share with the world.

Quitting the jungle juice is super important for everyone (I now believe) but quitting alcohol cold turkey can be dangerous due to potential withdrawal symptoms and medical complications. Seeking professional guidance and considering a structured approach to sobriety increases the likelihood of a safe and successful recovery.

The American Addictions Centre offers text or phone support. If you are needing text support please go to their website at americanaddictioncenters.org and fill in the form. The number that they have listed is (313) 214-2834 which can be used to access guidance about how to manage a medically managed detox which can ease the symptoms. They do state on their website "For those with alcohol dependence, quitting is not without risks. Acute alcohol withdrawal may be associated with certain medical complications. At American Addiction Centers (AAC), we offer 24-hour supervision and care during medical detox. We can help you get through the withdrawal process safely and with the aid of medical professionals."

Canada has a very extensive program through the www.canadadrugrehab.ca. Their phone number is 1.888.245.6887.

You can also fill out the form with your province and they will direct you to the appropriate resources.

I strongly encourage anyone facing a dependency on alcohol to reach out to a professional for help.

Drinking Responsibly

If you are able to (which I'm guessing you are not) drink responsibly then my hat goes off to you and I commend you. Moderation is a key aspect of maintaining a healthy and balanced lifestyle. It involves making conscious and mindful choices about alcohol consumption to ensure both personal well-being and the safety of others. Here's my comprehensive guide to drinking responsibly:

Understanding Responsible Drinking: The stuff they don't teach us in school.

1. Know Your Limits.

Be aware of your tolerance level and know when to stop drinking to avoid over consumption. According to Health Canada at www.canada.ca/en/health-canada/services/substance-use/alcohol/low-risk-alcohol-drinking-guidelines.
html these are the recommended levels for safer consumption of alcohol for women with the following being a "standard drink." In Canada, a standard drink is 17.05 millilitres or 13.45 grams of pure alcohol. This is the equivalent of:

- a bottle of beer (12 oz., 341 ml, 5% alcohol)
- a bottle of cider (12 oz., 341 ml, 5% alcohol)
- a glass of wine (5 oz., 142 ml, 12% alcohol)
- a shot glass of spirits (1.5 oz., 43 ml, 40% alcohol)

limit alcohol to no more than:

- 2 standard drinks per day
- 10 standard drinks per week

- 3 standard drinks on special occasions
- avoid drinking alcohol on some days

2. Know the Legal Drinking Age.

Abide by the legal drinking age in your location.

3. Educate Yourself.

Understand the standard drink measurements and alcohol content in various beverages if moderation is your modus operandi. Sometimes having a predetermined amount of consumption to maximally consume, may help. For me, that would never work as we know my addictive tendencies would kick in after the first glass.

Setting Boundaries

4. Plan Ahead.

Decide in advance how much you plan to drink and stick to your limit.

This is definitely easier said than done. I commend those who are able to do this.

5. Alternate with Water.

Intersperse alcoholic beverages with water to stay hydrated and pace yourself. Although if you have a problem with alcohol then you may just use this as a trick or tool in your arsenal to justify your drinking habits. I'm here to tell you that one glass of water does not negate one glass of booze.

6. Eat Before Drinking.

Consume a meal before drinking to slow down the absorption of alcohol into your bloodstream.

Even though we know we get wasted faster on an empty stomach and can generally drink less on an empty stomach to achieve the same result, having food prior to drinking does not negate the negative effects of drinking poison.

7. Avoid Binge Drinking.

Binge drinking, defined as consuming large amounts of alcohol in a short period, is associated with serious health risks. Avoid this! According to the center for disease control and prevention "binge drinking is defined as consuming 5 or more drinks on an occasion for men or 4 or more drinks on an occasion for women."
www.cdc.gov/alcohol/fact-sheets/binge-drinking.

Putting this into perspective for me... If one standard glass of wine is 5oz and there's 25oz in a bottle of wine then on average with my two bottles a night I was increasing my "recommended" booze intake by well over 100% each time I drank. Gross!

Responsible Behavior

8. Never Drink and Drive.

As we know, one of the most crucial aspects of responsible drinking is never driving under the influence. Arrange for a designated driver, use public transportation, or utilize rideshare services. Where I live we have a really neat service called Keys Please. I've used them more times than I'd like to admit – but so glad I did. Two people drive to your location in one vehicle then one person drives your vehicle with you in it home. It's a bit more expensive than a taxi but TOTALLY worth it. There's nothing worse than having to pick up your vehicle the morning after the night before. Feeling like shit, regretful and broke, hitting the McDonald's on the way if you can manage the anxiety and feeling of impending doom at the drive through window to get temporary relief for the incredible hunger. But that only lasts so long until you shit your brains out.

9. Be Mindful of Medications.

Check for interactions between alcohol and any medications you may be taking. Some medications can have adverse effects when combined with alcohol.

10. Respect Others' Choices.

Understand and respect others' decisions not to drink or to drink in moderation. We get it in our heads that it's more fun to drink when others are getting drunk with us. When in reality misery loves company. "Oh, come on, just have a drink with me" or "Let me get you a drink."

Moving forward, "NO" is now a complete sentence. We have to respect each other's decisions not to drink, and support them in these decisions. To all of my friends over the years who I have encouraged to drink after you have told me, "No." I'm sorry.

Social Responsibility

11. Host Responsibly.

If hosting an event with alcohol, provide non-alcoholic options, monitor guests' consumption, and encourage responsible behavior. Have a phone number readily available for your guests to arrange a taxi, or better yet have transportation available. For example, I had a Christmas party a few weeks before my last drink and I made it clear on my event page on Facebook that drinking and driving would not be acceptable, where I also shared my contact for keys please. Many of my guests were happy to use the service, knowing that they wouldn't have to come back in the morning all hungover.

12. Intervene if Necessary.

If you notice someone exhibiting signs of alcohol poisoning or with severely impaired judgment, intervene and seek help immediately by calling 911 (or your local emergency line) and getting them to the hospital. I actually had to do this once for a friend. Getting your stomach pumped is not the epitome of a good time.

17. Quitting Cold Turkey VS Drinking Responsibly

Recognizing Signs of a Problem

13. Practice Self-Reflection.

Assess your own drinking habits and be honest with yourself about any concerns. I was 100% honest with the outside world about my drinking. I played it off with jokes: "I'm definitely an alcoholic, it runs in my family", "I am my father's daughter", "It's wine o'clock somewhere", or "I don't have a problem I just really like to drink. I love how it makes me feel." I verbalized this so much that I used these as a front to mask the truth.

14. Seek Help if Needed.

If you find it challenging to drink responsibly or if alcohol is negatively impacting your life, seek support from friends, family, or professionals. This is fucking hard to do. If you are like me then I'm assuming you are confident, driven and maybe somewhat entitled when it comes to alcohol – like you DESERVE it or something. The last thing you want to do is reach out and say that you have a problem. "Who? Me? Nah! I'm good. I get up every day, the kids are fed and dressed, the house is clean, I cooked, I went to work." Sure! You do all of those things every day, it's a lot and I'm proud of you but if you do all of those things every day and your mornings start off where you feel like shit then you have a drink mid afternoon to feel better – it's time to seek help. It's okay. Help is literally there for people like us because it works! People make an honorable living off of us lol. Have solace in this... You will gain a new non judgemental sounding board that will help you get on your feet.

If you're spending the money anyways, it might as well be for your well being rather than to alcohol empires.

You have already been in a long-term relationship with alcohol, why not try a shorter term relationship with someone who can help you in your divorce. Let's be honest. Alcohol cessation is 100% like a divorce. It's been with you for a while, costs money, makes you feel shitty and it sucks to let it go but in the end you KNOW in your heart it's the right decision. People go to counselors for divorce. It's okay! The only person judging this decision is you! You got this!

Special Considerations

15. Pregnancy and Alcohol
Just don't – EVER!

16. Health Conditions
Consult with a healthcare professional if you have health conditions that may be affected by alcohol consumption.

Legal Implications:

17. Know Local Laws.
Familiarize yourself with local laws regarding alcohol consumption and adhere to them. Going to jail isn't a super fun experience anytime, but when you are drunk it's game over.

Remember, responsible drinking isn't just about not drinking and driving as we have just learned. It's a personal commitment that involves being mindful of your own health, safety, and the well-being of others. It's about making informed choices, setting boundaries, and being aware of the potential consequences of alcohol consumption. When struggling with alcohol-related issues, seeking support from friends, family, or professionals is a responsible and commendable step.

I'm proud of you!

CHAPTER 18

Accountability

Accountability is a crucial aspect of maintaining sobriety, and it involves taking responsibility for your actions, choices, and well-being. As a '90s girl, navigating the journey of sobriety, several factors contribute to accountability:

1. Personal Responsibility

Acknowledge that you are responsible for your choices and actions related to sobriety. This includes being accountable for your commitment to staying sober and making positive changes in your life. Just like you have had to be accountable to eating healthy, studying for an exam, going to work, finishing school, anything in your life that you wanted to succeed at you had to remain accountable to get the task done, right? There's nothing different here.

2. Setting Clear Boundaries

Establish clear boundaries to protect your sobriety. This may involve avoiding certain environments, events, or relationships that could jeopardize your commitment to being alcohol-free. My boundaries may and should be different from yours. You may want zero alcohol around you. Meaning... you don't want your friends/family to drink in your presence. You won't pick up alcohol for your partner after work, or you may choose not to go to the pub to socialize with your friends. Whatever works for you to keep you physically and mentally healthy. For me. I'm so confident in my sobriety and have such a deep knowledge that this is where I'm at now in my life that I don't care if others drink around me. Some people in my life CAN drink responsibly. They CAN only have one or two glasses of wine with supper. Now, that's commendable. It's just not me.

3. Building a Support System

Surround yourself with a strong support system of friends, family, or fellow sober people who understand your journey and encourage your commitment. Don't have these types of people? Find them! Create your own Facebook group. They will come to you. I can promise you that there's hundreds, if not thousands who are also wanting to get sober and want a sober community of people around them.

4. Regular Self-Reflection

Engage in regular self-reflection to assess your progress, identify potential triggers, and recognize areas for personal growth. This self-awareness contributes to accountability. What this looks like for you will be different from what it looks like for me. We were all cut from a different cloth so there isn't going to be a one-size-fits-all approach here.

5. Seeking Professional Help

If needed, seek professional help from therapists, counselors, or support groups specialized in addiction recovery. Professionals can provide guidance and tools for maintaining accountability. I was seeing my counselor for over a year because of my relationship with John. We did do a few sessions together. These sessions were unrelated to alcohol (when actually hindsight is always 20/20 – the turmoil in our relationship was 100% directly related to alcohol use and abuse on both ends). I highly encourage counseling or therapy. I believe that everyone can benefit from it.

6. Creating a Sobriety Plan

Develop a comprehensive sobriety plan that outlines your goals, coping strategies, and potential challenges. This plan can serve as a road map for accountability. This is going to be a lot harder than "Don't drink" or "Dry January, February or March", etc. Like seriously, what is the game plan for staying sober?

My game plan is taking my accountability seriously. Letting down the walls of my problems, and unapologetically being authentic about the use and abuse while announcing my sobriety. Honestly it took me over a month to announce it on FB publicly. First it was John, then I would randomly throw in conversation to my mother-in-law and children with: "We haven't had one drop since we have been on this work trip." Then I went on to tell a few friends like my best friend Tori of course, then one of my closest drinking buddies (via text). Next I told the "world" on FB about my sobriety by sharing my tattoo and the meaning of it. I got a tattoo in Victoria BC of a broken chain on my forearm and my post was captioned with…

> "Finally unchained from the grips of my past and damn does it feel good!
>
> Freedom from toxic thoughts and behaviors.
>
> I've begun writing my first book – something that I've wanted to do for decades.
>
> 45,000 words so far in about 2 weeks. It's gonna be a gooder! It already is
>
> Go smash life today people and have the BEST day ever!!!
>
> Love ya'll"

To be honest, I felt uneasy posting that at first. How were people going to react? Am I going to lose some friends? I've always been known as a partier and how I loved my wine.

So let's unpack that for a sec.

#1 How are people going to react? Who gives a fuck?

#2 Am I going to lose some friends? Yeah, maybe, but I guess if I lose friends for making a healthy decision for my physical and mental well-being then I guess that's on them and not me. People will come and go in our lives. It's hard but it's okay.

#3 Being known for being a partier and always having a glass of wine in my hand? That is definitely NOT the legacy I want to leave for myself or my kids. If I continued on the path of alcohol use I know it would have led to my death. At my funeral to be known as a wino and for everyone to also know that it's wine that killed me doesn't sit right with me and I'm not up for it anymore.

What does your sobriety plan look like? It may start out with "writing in my journal, admitting I have a problem" or maybe you are over it and want to scream it on your socials that you have a problem and need help? Maybe you want to call a counselor? Whatever path you choose is okay. Don't be stuck on the order of your operations. Plans change. Expect them to. Just start with something. Anything.

7. Accountability to Others

Communicate your commitment to sobriety with those close to you. This not only reinforces your dedication but also allows others to support and hold you accountable. Even if it's just one person that's okay. We all start somewhere. You may be ashamed that you have a problem and don't want to tell everyone you know. Let's work on switching the thoughts from "I have a problem with my drinking" to "I have a solution about my drinking." Now, doesn't that sound so much better?

8. Owning Your Story

Embrace your journey and be open about your experiences with sobriety. Sharing your story not only helps reduce your negative stigma but also reinforces your commitment through transparency. You don't need to be proud of your story, but you need to be honest. That old cliche is valid. "The truth shall set you free."

Point end case – this book. I'm Free.

9. Learning from Setbacks

You are going to have setbacks at first. There's just no avoiding them. Don't beat yourself over it. We are used to saying. "1 step forward, 2 steps back" – let's change that to "One step back, two steps forward." A change in your thoughts can and will change your life. One of my favorite earth angels who is now in the spirit world, Dr. Wayne Dyer wrote a book called, *Change your thoughts, Change Your Life* and one of his famous quotes is "I believe if you change the way you look at things, the things you look at change." What does that mean though when it comes to alcohol and setbacks? "Fuck! I failed today! I had a drink" reframe that to "Fuck, yeah! I only had one drink today and not my usual two bottles." What a difference it makes to just change the way you look at things.

Accept that setbacks may occur, and view them as opportunities for growth rather than failures. Learn from these experiences and adjust your approach to reinforce accountability.

10. Cultivating Healthy Coping Mechanisms

Accountability=honesty. Now, honestly drinking alcohol isn't a healthy coping mechanism, and if you believe it is – it MAY only be a temporary coping mechanism. You know the truth, that's why you picked up this book. Alcohol can and may only be a temporary immediate fix but it leads to long-term problems. Identify and practice healthy coping mechanisms to deal with stress, anxiety, or other emotions that might trigger the desire to drink.

11. Celebrating Milestones

Acknowledge and celebrate milestones in your sobriety journey. This positive reinforcement boosts morale and reinforces your commitment to being sober and gives you more confidence to keep going. "One day at a time" seems really cliche to me. It may be a mantra for you but for me I feel like it puts a lot of pressure on me to "get to the next day" and sort of seems like I'm wishing my life away. To start living and being present in each and every single moment completely sober is the goal. Having a clear mind not influenced by alcohol is how to truly be present. Celebrate sober cooking! Celebrate watching a hockey game sober! Celebrate going to bed sober. Celebrate waking up without a headache! No matter how small the milestone may be – it's yours and yours alone. You get to own it! Celebrate it!

12. Educating Yourself:

"Knowledge is power" is the old adage. But I believe that it's the practical use of that knowledge that is the ultimate power. You can have all the knowledge in the world but if you don't apply it then it's useless.

American Author and Speaker Dale Carnegie's famous quote is: "Knowledge isn't power until it is applied."

Stay informed about the effects of alcohol, the benefits of sobriety, and the resources available for support. Knowledge empowers you to make informed decisions, which is a superpower.

13. Prioritizing Self-Care

Prioritize self-care activities that contribute to your overall well-being. This includes maintaining a healthy lifestyle, engaging in activities you enjoy, and getting enough rest. For the moms in the back, NO! This does not mean getting groceries by yourself without your kids. No, this does not mean you get to have a shower without children coming in. It means going to a bookstore and sitting for a few hours with a coffee and a good read. It means going to a yoga class THEN to the library to write in your journal. It means sitting by a river and just being by yourself for a couple hours. It means going for a walk and listening to audiobooks by yourself. It means not feeling guilty for doing you and doing what makes you happy. This might take some time to figure out what that is, especially when it was booze that made you happy. Prioritize yourself in order to be your best self. Only then can you be the woman, mother, spouse and friend you were meant to be. You can't give a dollar if you don't have a dollar. This, my friend, is a liberating statement.

14. Being Mindful of Triggers

Identifying and being mindful of situations, people, or emotions that may act as triggers for alcohol use will help you not to use. You need to develop strategies to navigate these triggers without compromising your sobriety. It's hard but worth it.

My situations? So I don't think that I could just stop cooking or cleaning altogether. Could you imagine? I'm a neat freak naturally (so much so that I own a cleaning business). To think of the state of my house if I were to just completely abolish the duties I set out for myself as a mother and a homeowner. Let's just say it would be just short of disastrous. Now that I'm home temporarily from the work trip that got me sober, I'm still cooking and cleaning – no problem. I'm probably cleaning even more to be honest. It keeps me busy. One thing I HAVE noticed is that I constantly have a drink in my hand, albeit it coffee, tea, flavored or fizzy anything such as Sanpellegrino, Bubbly, Guru (no I'm not a paid sponsor for these), etc. Water isn't cutting it, but I'm workin' on it.

I also love cooking for my family and seeing them eat up the creations I make. It makes me feel proud, happy and know that I'm doing a good job. The difference from when I was cooking before was that in my mind's eye there was only Netflix, wine and me. It was "my time."

But now… It's conversation, the babies helping (sometimes), laughing, dancing and me. I'm not secluding myself from my family as I cook for them. What has also changed is the fact that I now eat with those I cook for. I was always one of those "Can't eat until I'm done drinking" kinda people. That would often mean that I didn't eat until 1-2am or I would just have a disgusting carby snack OR I wouldn't eat the supper I made at all.

I would then order Indian food, pizza or Italian from some fancy schmancy restaurant. Although you would REALLY know if I was wasted if I got nachos or taquitos from the 7-11 loaded with cheese, sour cream, banana peppers, onions and their sweet ketchup sauce, then didn't actually eat it… Seeing it on my nightstand the next morning was a lovely reminder of my wasted night before.

My people? So many of the people I know and who I considered "friends" were people from the pub and/or the casino. I would tell John that I liked to go to the casino by myself because that's where my friends were. I laughed with them, I got drunk with them. I eventually got to "VIP" status lol. I never paid for a single drink. I guess that's what happens when you are throwing away tens of thousands of dollars placing $25-$250 bets on the slot machines. Or as I like to call them… The "slut" machines.

I loved to tip them well and just chat. They were the most expensive friends I've ever had.

I have my girlfriends who are my drinking buddies, where every single time we get together it's just a booze fest. Time to get some new friends I suppose.

Emotions? I don't think I was ever really an emotional drinker. I mean sure I'd have days when I would say "I need a drink." The last time I remember saying that was around Christmas time last year before I had to go see my mother. I would also have days here and there where I went for a cold beer after a long hot day working outside or gardening. Though I was never one who was like, "I'm sad, I need a drink, I'm feeling this or that and I need a drink." If I wasn't pregnant or working I had a drink in my hand.

15. Focusing on Personal Growth

Try viewing sobriety as an opportunity for personal growth. I believe it truly is. When you make the decision to become sober you literally decide to shed the old you and with this you automatically grow into a completely new and awakened person. How can you be the same person you were when you were drinking? Impossible. You can't. This new journey in sobriety is yours to use however you want. To start tackling that ever growing list of "things to do" that you kept putting off because drinking was more important. Use that time and energy previously spent on alcohol to invest in your passions, hobbies, and self-improvement. As you know, that time for me is now being more present with my children, and writing this damn book!

16. Staying Present

Practice mindfulness and staying present "in the moment." This can help you avoid dwelling on the past or worrying about the future, promoting a positive and accountable mindset.

17. Learning to Say "No"

I have gotten to a point now where I'm super comfortable saying "No" to events and/or people where the premise is "Let's get wasted." I did that for over 20 years. I know what it's about and I'm confident in my decision not to be that person anymore.

It may take time for you to gain that confidence though. How do you find that confidence? Well, to be honest, I feel like that may look different for everyone. For me it was just sticking to my guns and knowing that it gets easier to say, "No." Once you have mastered saying "No" to yourself, you can say "No" to anyone! Be comfortable saying "no" to situations or invitations that may compromise your sobriety. Assertiveness is going to be a key aspect of accountability.

18. Routine Check-Ins

Regularly check in with yourself and assess your emotional and mental well-being. This self-awareness aids in maintaining accountability.

"Knock knock. Who's there? Sober Challaine. Sober Challaine who? You know, the real you who quit drinking poison and are now living your best life ever?"

If you have to say something stupid to yourself like that then by all means, why not? Check in, do an inventory on your life every day. Write about it, talk to yourself about what's going on. What struggles are you facing? What accomplishments are you facing? How has being sober changed you? How has it not changed you? What goals are you accomplishing? All of these are super important to help keep you on track. It can serve as a mental road map (or physical if you chose to write it down) of where you came from to where you are today. Try to highlight the positive changes. Emphasize the positive aspects of your decision, such as improved health, mental clarity, and personal growth. Make it clear to yourself that sobriety is a choice you've made for your well-being. Don't expect it to be linear! You are setting yourself up for failure if this is your belief. Most trajectories in life are not linear at all and there are going to be bumps in the road. You need to keep on keepin' on. You will realize that after every bump they end up in the rear view.

19. Engaging in Sober Activities

Explore and engage in activities that align with your sober lifestyle. This can include sober events, hobbies, or new experiences that contribute to your overall happiness. Easier said than done. I know what you're thinking: "Challaine I've been an alcoholic for x amount of years. All of my activities revolve around booze. All of my friends drink."

I hear you and I can 100% empathize with you. I get it, I understand. Although, the mother in me is going to tell you, "Tough luck, kid. Get new friends and get a new hobby." Sorry if that sounds a little harsh although we are all grown ups here and can handle the cold hard truth. How in the hell can you expect to change your life if you don't change the circumstances in your life? Impossible.

If you are completely terrified of change and are such a creature of habit (I am to the latter one) then take it slow. However, keep in mind though, the slower you move in building a new life for yourself the longer it's going to take to build the life of your dreams.

20. Continual Growth and Adaptation

Sobriety is a journey of continual growth and adaptation. Be open to evolving strategies, seeking new insights, and adjusting your approach as needed.

Remember, accountability is a dynamic and ongoing process. By being proactive, staying connected to your support system, and prioritizing your well-being, you can successfully navigate the challenges of sobriety. With accountability, it's nice to be able to have our friends' continued support. To be honest though, you may lose some friendships through your authentic journey. Especially the friends you used to drink with or party with. This can be a huge adjustment for both of you. There may be resentment on both sides. People tend to get uncomfortable, defensive and angry when they see someone they love start to outgrow them in a relationship. These relationships can mean your friends, spouse, family, co-workers. Literally anyone you have a "relationship" with. You need to put yourself first though. You have made the decision to live your life healthy, happy and free from the ball and chain that is attached to the bottle and your hand so if you lose some people along the way, it's going to be hard but it's going to be okay.

There are a few ways to navigate the reactions of your friends who don't support your journey. If there's resistance with their acceptance (which you don't need by the way, in order to succeed) then talk with them. Try to get to the root of what they are going through and why they are offended that you are changing your life. Sounds weird when I lay it out like that, right?

If your friends chose not to support you or hang out with you anymore remember it has nothing to do with you and everything to do with them. They are either too embarrassed to admit they have a problem and can't socialize with you sober or you have become an unintentional threat and you just outshine them now and that makes them super uncomfortable because maybe they have always been the star of the show?

Or… Perhaps they want to become sober too and just aren't ready yet. That's okay. Just like those in my life the past couple of years wanted me to get sober, I couldn't and wouldn't until I wanted to.

Offer your support and be open to any questions they may have but don't shove your sobriety in their face. It's kind of like that old joke "How do you know there is a gluten free vegetarian in the room? Don't worry they will tell you." We all know that one person and it's super annoying, right? Don't be that person. In my opinion.

Yes! Own your sobriety but it doesn't have to be the main topic of conversation when you see someone. If you have boundaries about being around other people drinking then that needs to be discussed for sure. For me, I don't give a fuck if you want to have a drink or three around me. I'm not going to cave or give in. I'm so right in my head now that I'm not tempted.

Talking to friends about your decision to be sober can be a significant step in your journey towards a healthier lifestyle. Here are some tips to help you approach this conversation:

1. Choose the Right Setting.

I'm not going to tell you to find a quiet and comfortable setting where you can have an open and honest conversation without distractions. That would be super awkward for me and my friends if I brought them to the library and sat in a pow wow circle on the carpet to discuss my sobriety. Not for me. What are you comfortable with?

Are you more comfortable to chat over text? Do it!

On the phone? Do it!

In person? Do it!

Carrier pigeon? Do it!

Snail mail? Do it!

Let the whole world know at once on social media? Do it!

For me it was a one on one basis over text, then I did the whole social media thing.

I have found with social media – those who are moving through sobriety or are sober will like your posts more than those who are not. Interesting how it worked out that way. Nobody that I used to drink with "supports me" or "likes" any of my sobriety posts. Perhaps it's making them question their relationship with alcohol? It goes both ways I suppose. I no longer like posts from my friends where they are holding a drink or posting memes about alcohol. The difference between them and me is that I've already questioned my relationship with alcohol and know the answer. I hope that I can be an inspiration to my friends and family while also being a support if they need it.

Wherever or however you choose to do it, just be honest and open. There's no right way or wrong way. Approach the conversation with honesty. Share your feelings, experiences, and the reasons behind your decision to be sober. If you want. Let your friends know that you trust and value their support. It may help guide them in their new role to being a friend for you. Some people need that type of direction, others don't.

You will hopefully know your friends best and can make the best decision for you.

2. Use "I" Statements.

Frame your conversations using "I" statements to express your feelings and decisions without placing blame. For example, say "I have decided to be sober because..." instead of "You make me want to quit drinking." That's that whole accountability thing. Sure others may influence your desire to quit, but you need to quit and make an impact on yourself before it will impact others.

You getting sober has nothing to do with everyone and everything to do with you. I know you might be saying to yourself "Challaine, I need to get sober for my family." You see in that sentence that "I" comes before family? Sit with that for a minute.

Ur welcome ;)

3 Express Gratitude for Their Friendship.

You got to a place in your friendships because of "something." What is that something? Is it deeper than alcohol? If you believe it is, find it, talk about it and start with that. Let your friends know how much you value their friendship and support and thank them for being there. Acknowledge any positive experiences you've shared while being on your journey while also explaining why sobriety is essential for you at this point in your life. If they are boozers. What is their take on getting sober for them? How can you help?

4. Set Boundaries.

This is a repeated statement to living a sober life. You HAVE to clearly communicate any boundaries related to your sobriety with those around you. This may include avoiding certain environments or events where alcohol is prevalent. Be firm but respectful in expressing your needs. Your needs are just as important as others.

5. Be Prepared for Various Reactions.

Understand that your friends may have different reactions. Some may be supportive and understanding, while others might be doubtful or may need time to process the information. Have you told people before that you have stopped drinking? The majority of people do not get sober on their first attempt so your people might think you are full of shit – just like last time. I'm pretty sure I couldn't even count the amount of times I was going to quit drinking. Be patient and allow them the space to react. My circle has been super supportive and for that I'm incredibly grateful.

My oldest son, though, was really hesitant at first and didn't believe me this time. I've broken my promise to him on more than one occasion. He said something along the lines of "Yeah, until something happens and you need a drink." I was able to look at him confidently and tell him that, "No, I'm done." He felt awkward, which is his to own and process, but I felt great owning my answer and having the confidence to know in my heart that it was true this time…

6. Offer Reassurance.

Reassure your friends that your decision to be sober is about your personal growth and well-being, not a judgment on their choices. Make it clear that you still value and respect their decisions. This is super important, especially for the friends that have been with you for a while and who may have been your drinking buddies. Maybe these friends only drank socially and were able to stop. Maybe these friends don't have a problem with alcohol and are able to "drink responsibly." The choice to get sober is a choice for you. Just like you will do it on your own time so will others, if they choose. Just because you decided to get sober it doesn't change your love for anyone who continues to drink. It may (or may not) however, put up some boundaries in regards to what you allow in your life or around you.

7. Provide Resources.

If your friends express interest in learning more about addiction or sobriety, offer them resources or recommend educational materials. This can help them better understand your perspective. Hint, hint – nudge nudge… This book!

You may not have all the answers for what someone else may be looking for but be open to help find them and offer up resources that have worked for you.

8. Ask for Support.

Clearly communicate how your friends can support you in your journey. Whether it's providing encouragement, participating in sober activities (if they are comfortable going with you), or being understanding in certain situations, let them know what you need.

9. Stay Calm and Patient.

Be prepared for a range of emotions from your friends. Stay calm, patient, and open to further discussions. Allow them time to process the information and ask questions.

10. Invite Them to Join in Sober Activities.

If appropriate, invite your friends to participate in activities that don't involve alcohol. Show them that your decision to be sober doesn't mean the end of your social life but rather a shift towards healthier alternatives. This may be completely awkward at first. The first sober hang out I had with my ex-neighbor friends was really weird for the first half hour or so as it was seriously like the first time in almost seven years that we had hung out and weren't drinking together. After the first little bit we found a new groove. Lucky for us they are on the same page as us as far as ditching the booze train.

11. Follow Up.

Check in with your friends periodically to update them on your progress and to check on them too. Sharing your achievements and challenges will help reinforce the importance of their support. This goes two ways though. Don't use your sobriety to put other people down. Unintentionally of course, although you need to be mindful. If you have peers going through a similar journey, hear them out. Talk about them first. Maybe they have had a really hard day and couldn't stay away from the booze, now would not be a good time to go on about your achievements for today. As you may know… This will just make them feel shittier about themselves. Be a leader… If you stay strong while being supportive that may be all that someone else needs to help them. You literally have the power to save someone's life. Now, THAT'S a big deal!

12. Seek Professional Guidance if Necessary.
If you anticipate significant challenges in discussing your sobriety with certain friends or family members, or if you're concerned about their reactions, consider seeking advice from a therapist or counselor.

Remember, everyone's journey is unique, and your friends may respond differently than what you had anticipated. Be patient and understanding, and surround yourself with those who offer support and encouragement on your path to sobriety.

My counselor has been amazing for me. Was it her that made me quit? No, not specifically. I believe it was a culmination of my expressions with her, my own demise and her understanding while being empathetic to the chaos in my life that helped get me to where I am now.

Therapy may or may not be for you. You can't decide that it's not though, until you try. I'm not talking about one session. You could have one session with someone who isn't a good fit. It's a relationship. Don't forget that. I encourage you to try a minimum of three different therapists and go to at least three sessions with one that is a good fit before you decide that therapy is not for you.

You may be pleasantly surprised though what you get out of your sessions. With every layer peeled back and raw emotion that comes out – the authentic you has a chance to shine. Give yourself the chance.

Shine.

CHAPTER 19

Lessons Learned

Navigate a future without alcohol. Can you even picture it? If you haven't quit yet, you probably can't imagine a life without alcohol, or maybe you can but it's a little fuzzy or unclear. If you are this far into my book you have either really started contemplating it or are on your way and this has been a support tool for you. If it's the latter I'm so happy to have been able to be a part of your journey. Thank you.

As you embark on the road ahead towards a future without alcohol, envisioning the chapters of this sober life can be both exhilarating and transformative but questionable. In the following exploration, we dive into the vast expanse of possibilities, challenges, and profound revelations that await on the horizon of a life liberated from the chains of alcohol.

1. The Blank Canvas: A Fresh Start

Embracing New Beginnings
Blank.
  New.
  Beginnings.
  Look at all of the opportunities that lie in those three words alone. Absolutely incredible if I do say so myself.
  How often do we get to start over? Rebirth? Become someone new? Usually it takes something incredibly significant in our lives that will allow us the opportunity to make this happen... Becoming a parent, graduating, losing a loved one,

getting married, a near death experience, getting sober. What instances in life do you correlate with rebirth?

Starting over and shedding the old you can be scary. You, as you know it, is all you have ever known. How the fuck are you supposed to navigate this world without your crutch?

When my dad died, I lost my best friend. It was hard. It is still hard. I miss him every single day. I see him show up in littles hints throughout my day. I feel him throughout my day. But he's gone and that's a fact. My life is completely different without him around. It's hard but I'm adapting and I'm getting by.

Same without having alcohol in my life. I've been really tested the past few weeks with my sobriety and the stress of my life. I was robbed twice in the same month. I was fucking mad at the world. I was mad at God. I was mad at my dad for not protecting me and guiding me. I was just fucking mad. The old habitual drinker in me that still kind of pops in here and there was REALLY tempted to get wine (one day in particular). I didn't though because that old me doesn't exist anymore. Literally. I'm physically and mentally unable to connect alcohol to my new mind and way of thinking with my new body being alcohol free. Self positive talk got me out of it. I guess I sort of have a fear of alcohol now. A fear of who I will become if I drink, a fear of not being able to only have one, the fear of being hungover, the fear of spending money, the fear of doing something stupid, the fear of fighting with John. Generally, if you are scared of something then you probably shouldn't do it. I just don't. It's not worth the fear, and plus I've been drunk enough to know that the results are ALWAYS the same.

The decision to live a future without alcohol can mark a poignant moment of rebirth. I want you to picture two blank canvases stretched before you. Canvas #1 is waiting to be adorned with the vibrant strokes of a life crafted with intention and sobriety. Canvas #2 is a canvas adorned with the events of the past while alcohol was present. #1 is free, clear, ambitious, adventurous, shame and guilt free. While #2 I'm willing to bet has a feeling attached to it that is sticky, uncomfortable, scary, uneasy. Either canvas you choose is a choice, choose wisely.

Rediscovering Self-Identity

As the echoes of alcohol fade into the background over time, the opportunity for self-discovery unfolds. Embrace the chance to redefine your identity, rediscover passions, and reconnect with the authentic essence of who you are. I don't want you to negate or invalidate your relationship with your past. It got you to this point. If you can get through all that bull shit and finally put the bottle down then you can do anything. You can count your echoes in seconds, minutes, hours, days, years… Do whatever you need to do to know that it's in the past and is staying there. If "I've been sober for 72 hours" FEELS longer to you and gives you a greater sense of accomplishment than "I've been sober for three days" then go with whatever makes you FEEL most powerful. You are in control now. Own it. Create your new journey.

Setting Purposeful Intentions

In this blank canvas of your future, set intentions with purpose. What the fuck are you going to do with your life now that you aren't a fucking drunk? What are you going to do with your extra time? Your extra money? Your extra energy? I'm a list person. Write a list for all of these things. A list of intentions. Your list doesn't have to be gargantuan. I mean it can be but it doesn't have to. Here's just a little sample list for me.

- Extra money – pay off the gambling debt and save, not eat so much take out.
- Extra time – I won't be hungover anymore in the mornings, so I will have time to write and get office work done.
- Extra energy – I will have the energy to go to the gym with my daughter.

- More Goals – To write my book and publish it for the world. To help people through my sobriety initiatives.

Envision the person you aspire to become, the relationships you aim to cultivate, and the legacy you wish to leave. Every brushstroke is a conscious step towards a life aligned with your values.

2. A Tapestry of Health and Wellness

Physical Well-Being
Picture the future as a tapestry woven with threads of enhanced physical well-being. Freed from the detrimental effects of alcohol, your body undergoes a revitalization. Visualize a life brimming with energy, vitality, and the joy of a healthy, well-nourished existence. Remember when we were younger and could drink until 4 am, sleep for three hours and be ready for work for 9am and actually talk to people? FYI, in case you didn't know, you are NOT that person anymore. Part of the reason why you can't do that anymore is age and the fact that you have destroyed your body from the effects of alcohol. You have stripped your body of the essential vitamins and minerals that aid in the natural processes of detoxifying and healing. We are meant to detoxify impurities in small doses like a bit of car exhaust here and there, inorganic food, etc. Not gallons and gallons of poisonous alcohol. Kudos to our bodies for putting up with so much and detoxifying us when we needed it, but it's tired now. It's time to rejuvenate and re energize and rebirth.

Mental Clarity and Emotional Resilience
As sobriety becomes a cornerstone of your future, envision mental clarity and emotional resilience emerging as your allies. You don't NEED alcohol to be there for you anymore. In all honesty, was it really ever there for you? Alcohol wasn't and isn't an ally. It was merely just an enemy just masked as an ally

19. Lessons Learned

but in reality just fucked you without lube and never apologized for being a fake ass friend.

You are perfect just the way you are without the influence of booze. Picture a mind unburdened by the fog of substances, capable of navigating life's challenges with grace and fortitude.

Can you picture that? No?

Try!

Still can't?

Try again!

Keep trying until you can see it. Hold that vision, even if it's just for a minute. I want you to FEEL what living with a clear mind is like. Pretend it's already there. Don't lose your focus until it becomes your reality. You have convinced yourself for long enough that alcohol was okay in your life. It's now time to convince yourself, until it becomes your truth, that it's not okay in your life!

Think this is all hog wash? Try this then. Have you ever planned a vacation or planned a date? You know that feeling of excitement and being giddy? THAT! That right there is the feeling that we are going for. The vacation or date hasn't happened yet but you can FEEL what it's going to be like because you can picture it.

I don't expect you to get it right the first time, or even the second or third. Just keep going! Picture and feel your life unchained.

Holistic Wellness Practices

Imagine incorporating holistic wellness practices into your daily routine. Or don't. The choice is ultimately yours. You will never know what works for you though, unless you try, right?

You can try anything from mindfulness and meditation to nourishing nutrition and regular exercise, visualize a future where your well-being is prioritized in every aspect of your life.

3. Fulfilling Relationships

Building Authentic Connections

How many of your relationships or friendships are authentic? I'm going to just speculate that you say "all of them." I would like to challenge that with a simple task. I want you to associate or hang out with the people that you drink with but now.... without alcohol. What do you have in common? What do you talk about? What do you do? Is it awkward? I want you to really evaluate the authenticity of not just those around you but YOU with those around you. I think you will be surprised, maybe even hurt to know that it wasn't all that it was made out to be. That's okay... It's your time now. You get to choose the quality of your life now and who you get to share your precious time with. We are only here for a short while, so we might as well make it worth it.

As the specter of alcohol dissipates, envision a future adorned with authentic connections. Cultivate relationships based on shared values, mutual respect, and genuine understanding. Picture the joy of bonding with others on a deeper, more meaningful level.

Nurturing Family Ties

I'm working on that one. It's been almost two months of complete sobriety. Not one drop and my 12 year old still doesn't believe me. She brought up to me tonight how I lied to NiK for a few birthdays that I wouldn't drink and never kept my promises. I showed her my tattoo of my broken chains. She called my tattoo stupid, lol. I have a lot of proving to my kids to do. I can't erase the hurt from the past but I can do better for our future.

I need to work on visualizing the profound impact of sobriety on my family relationships. Picturing the moments of shared laughter, the strength of unity during challenges, and the deepening of bonds as we navigate the journey of life together. I challenge you to do the same.

19. Lessons Learned

Socializing Without Substances

Is that even possible? In a world where it's thrown at us as the only means to have fun, it certainly seems impossible.

Awkward? Yes.

Only at first though.

Impossible? No.

You are going to have a sense or feeling of knowing this to be true and I bet you are going to avoid your friends, maybe even your family as you first enter your sobriety because you won't know how to "act" around them. You aren't going to be sure on how to project the new "you." The "authentic" you. I mean, fuck! How the hell are you supposed to share this new you if you don't even know who this new you is yet?

Remember how we talked about moving "through." Here's another instance:

You will feel the resistance but you need to push through the uncomfortable in order to get comfortable. They will be getting to know the new you WITH you. What harm can be done in that? I mean you never know unless you try, right?

I suggest trying something new altogether. If you and your friends always go to the local bar and get wasted, I wouldn't recommend going to that bar and everyone not drink. Just writing that sounds weird and uncomfortable. Maybe that bar will be left in the rearview with the memories and you can find a new hangout spot that isn't attached to the alcohol.

I used to always go to our local pub "Bogey's." Like the casino, it was where my "friends" were. What a lie. Of course people are going to be friendly when you spend money (thousands on VLTs) and drink the bar almost dry.

I quit going to Bogey's long before I got sober. I don't have any reason to go there anymore. It was my dad's bar that he would frequent every day. John and I would go there every night after work before we became obsessed with the casino. When I think about it now I just feel uncomfortable, regretful for spending so much time and money there. What was it all for? Expensive drinks, the thrill of pushing a button and losing, or I guess chasing the little wins here and there, seeing the familiar faces.

It's hard to let the past go I suppose. For whatever reason those years were a part of my life for reasons, some unbeknownst to me.

We need to envision a social landscape free of alcohol. Picture gatherings infused with genuine connection, where laughter flows naturally, and the joy of shared experiences takes center stage. Seeing ourselves navigating social situations confidently and authentically. It'll take time as the familiar is comfortable. But remember …. Just like any intimate relationship, when you know it's over and you become roommates, it's hard to let go but it's necessary. It's okay to say "Goodbye" to social circles and events where alcohol was so prevalent. You are building a new life now. So am I.

4. Professional Growth and Fulfillment

Career Ambitions Unleashed

Let's be honest. Are you really thriving at your job/career as a drunk? I thought I was. I thought I had all my poop in a group. "I own two businesses, have four kids, and, and, and…"

How can you grow, expand, produce, think clearly with a poisoned and exhausted mind? You can't. Why? Because you're exhausted. Simple.

How often have you pushed off tasks that were mandatory but somehow you weaseled your way into getting out of them? Both hands way up for me! I don't even know how I pulled some of those hungover days off. My only explanation is miracles.

Can you picture a work environment where productivity and focus are your steadfast companions? Now THAT would be a miracle, wouldn't it? Freed from the distractions of alcohol in the workplace or going for drinks after work. Freed from the terrible morning after the night before and having to face your

19. Lessons Learned

coworkers. Visualize yourself excelling in your endeavors, making significant contributions, and reaching new heights in your professional journey. Imagine what impact you would have if you showed up to work happy because you weren't filled with poison? You being sober could in reality affect so many other people in such a positive way, which could ripple into the company you work for, benefiting them as well, which is just a win-win all around.

Imagine the entrepreneurial ventures and creative endeavors that flourish in the soil of a sober mind. Picture yourself tapping into newfound creativity, exploring innovative ideas, and bringing your passions to life with a clarity of purpose. Imagine if you were always quiet and hungover in the corner, and now you're not. Your imagination has come to life and you get to share that with everyone around you. Bring yourself professionally to new heights.

What are your goals and dreams? Even if you haven't become sober yet. What are they? Whatever they are – they are IMPORTANT, and they matter! Why? Because you are important and you matter. If you didn't you wouldn't have been born. Plain and simple. Everyone on this planet – even if we can't pinpoint it at any given time – has a purpose.

It's often during the sticky times in our lives when we begin to question our purpose or even our existence. I know I have. I am right now as I put this book together. I've had many jobs/careers in my life and always thought those were my purpose, my calling. Over the years my calling has changed, several times to be honest. It's changing now and you are a part of this with me.

I've always wanted to write a book. I knew I had something to say, but never knew what to say. I guess 10 years ago when I was in the fun of the drinking and living my life as a fit Personal Trainer, I just didn't have enough trauma or experience to write anything of real significance.

Here we go again – I had to go THROUGH all of that shit to bring me here, to write this for you, for me. See how this going "through" keeps coming around?

What is the purpose of this book? What's my goal? Well, I've always been one that people/clients looked up to (although I hid my dirty little secrets pretty well from them), and being in a "position of authority" or "the boss" as a business owner. I feel that with writing this book and sharing my story, I will get into coaching again and helping people is my calling at this phase in my life. I'm committed to be of service to others, whatever that may look like.

Who knows? Maybe I will write ten more books and be a nutty old lady in her office writing until she dies. Maybe I'll switch gears again and become a skydiving instructor (highly unlikely but I remain open). I will be someone new in ten years and this awakening will just be another blip in time. Even though it's so significant now.

Wow, it's so weird. Just a blip.

Bottom line is I love to help people, I love to give, I love to make a positive impact on anyone if I'm able to.

To be able to do these things, and reach these goals of impacting as many lives as possible I have to keep pushing through. So you (unknowingly) hold me accountable, where in turn I can hold you accountable and be there for you.

As you gaze into the future, see your career aspirations taking flight. Sobriety becomes a catalyst for professional growth, unlocking your full potential and allowing you to pursue your passions with unwavering focus and dedication.

If I didn't have this audience that I wanted to reach I wouldn't be well on my new path and/or would probably still be drinking. There's this little voice inside me though that keeps saying "don't lie to them, don't let them down."

If it's not for yourself then who are you not going to lie to or let down? Sometimes having that person in your mind is all you need to stay on track.

I have zero guarantees that I will ever sell one copy of this book. I mean I hope that's not the case of course but knowing that the potential is there in order to dump some good shit in this world will keep me on the yellow brick road.

So if I sell even one, thank you. Mission complete.

5. Personal Growth and Continuous Learning

Lifelong Learning

"When the Student is ready the Teacher will appear."

– Lao Tzu.

"You will continue to be taught the lesson until the lesson is learned."

– Me.

I'm sure someone else was quoted for saying that but I'm not sure who is, although I know I say it all the time.

Are you ever fucking sick of being taught the same lesson over and over again? Like how many damn times did I have to be taught that drinking is a terrible idea, that gambling is a terrible idea? Why couldn't I have had my **Brain Wow** moment of *I Just Woke Up One Day & Changed My F*cking Mind* say like ten years ago?

I may never fully know that answer, but I am grateful that it has brought me here and now. I am grateful that my older children are witnessing their mother being sober, even though it's still sort of weird for them. I'm grateful that my lesson was finally learned before my babies witnessed the chaos of my drunk ass, and have those memories imprinted in their minds for the rest of their lives.

I am grateful that my previous existence on this earth and all the dumb shit that I did got me to this point – to finally write my book.

I am grateful. I have learned a LOT about myself during this whole process. Looking back over the past twenty years, the past two years, the past two months.

We will all be students of life. No matter how hard we try to fight it and try to get things done on our own time (the one that our ego decides). Sometimes we just have to ride through the waves until divine order glides us into shore exactly where we need to be. Me writing this book. You reading this book.

I'm empowered to continue my vision for a future marked by continuous personal growth and a thirst for knowledge. I'm excited to picture myself as a lifelong learner, exploring new interests, acquiring skills, and expanding my horizons in a world brimming with opportunities.

What are your goals for your personal life? What do you want to learn about yourself? What do you want to learn about in general? It's true that the world is our oyster. We tend to get so confined in the preconditioning of what others tell us or what we tell ourselves. What we are and aren't capable of doing. With a clear mind free from alcohol and the shitty lifestyle it leads there are so many opportunities that await us.

I absolutely love vision boards! Create one. Don't know where to start? Google it for inspiration! It's really quite simple. If you can think about it, if you can visualize it then you can achieve it. They have apps now where you can create a vision board in your phone so it's always with you. I like the idea of a huge vision board on the wall in my office. I remember back in the day when I would cut out magazine pictures and words to put on my vision boards. It's fun, it's crafty and creative. If this is your jam, I encourage you to do it that way.

Resilience in the Face of Challenges

As you navigate the terrain of your future, visualize the resilience cultivated through sobriety. Think of everything in your past that hasn't been easy. Did you make it? Barely? Every other possibility is accurate except for "no." You know how I know that? Because you are here! You persevered. You freakin'

19. Lessons Learned

made it! Now keep going! There's going to be tens if not hundreds of more challenges as we continue spinning around in this universe. The past may be behind us but it got us here.

Envision a future where self-improvement is a continuous journey, and each experience becomes a stepping stone towards becoming the best version of yourself. Picture yourself facing any challenge with a sense of equanimity, turning obstacles into opportunities for personal evolution.

Don't.

Fucking.

Quit.

6. Financial Stability and Freedom

Responsible Financial Choices

Can you picture a future characterized by responsible financial choices? Sounds interesting doesn't it?

What? No more spending $150 a night on copious amounts of Indian food (my absolutely fave "I'm wasted" food), $60 a night on booze plus a pack of smokes, thousands of dollars on VLTs and hundreds on "Keys Please Sober Drivers. Ugh… writing it all out makes me sick. Although that was my reality I apparently need to be reminded of it in order to keep my mental ducks in a row and to reaffirm that I do NOT want to live that lifestyle anymore. I'm getting too fucking old for this shit. If I didn't drink and gamble my life away I would be a fucking millionaire by now. K well I didn't gamble my WHOLE life away. But you know what I mean.

How do you spend frivolously when you drink? What are your dirty habits? Can you tally up your list of all the stupid shit that you buy while drinking (including the booze), what does your Amazon checkout history look like? What does that yearly total look like? Not sure? Get honest with yourself. Open up your banking app. Check out the last month.

Go!

Go do it!

I'll wait.

A couple hundred? Thousand a month? Multiply that by twelve. How does it make you feel? Pretty shitty I suppose.

Now try this... Take that exact same number and make a list of what you could spend that money on instead? Savings? Vehicle or home repairs, therapy, vacation.

What's your number? What are you going to do with all that money now?

My number.... It's A LOT. Definitely upwards of $200,000 a year.

You know how much shit I'm going to get done with $200,000 now?

I'm so excited for what this new year is going to bring me in regards to my finances as I'm literally not pissing them down the drain anymore. In the most literal sense.

Sobriety can empower us to allocate resources wisely, make informed decisions, and build a foundation of financial stability that affords us greater freedom and security. Doesn't that sound fun?

I can visualize myself pursuing and achieving financial goals with determination. It's fucking go time, cuz my go time is going to be gone time if I don't put some pep in my step!

Can you picture the satisfaction that comes from aligning your financial endeavors with your values and aspirations, creating a life of purpose and abundance? I certainly can.

As I peer into my future, I see the liberation from the financial burden of alcohol abuse and habit. Sobriety opens the door to a world where resources are directed towards meaningful pursuits, unencumbered by the weight of substances.

Ahhhhh, what a load is lifted.

7. Community Involvement and Giving Back:

Envision a future where community involvement becomes a cornerstone of your life. Picture yourself contributing to causes that resonate with your values, actively participating in community initiatives, and making a positive impact on the lives of those around you.

8. Travel and Exploration

Sober Adventures

Vacation and traveling always meant "LET'S GET WASTED!" Even on work trips. Literally every single vacation I have been on I've been wasted. Puking on top of the Eiffel Tower, drunken horseback riding in Mexico. Have you ever tried to puke while vertical in the ocean wearing a life jacket? I have and it was terrible. One of the worst hangovers of my life. After that debauchery, we took the boat back, got off and started walking up the pier back to land. I puked again, INTO the wind... Fucking Gross...Yeah, that was absolutely not one of my most proudest moments. Enough said.

I literally don't have any memories of a sober vacation.

Oh, wait! That's a lie. When I was a nanny, I went to Mexico and Florida with the family. I was sober (I was working). That's one thing I've never done was work while drunk.

What memories do you have of vacation? Similar to mine? If so, it's time to change that.

Let's create our world of sober adventures that await us. Picture the thrill of exploring new cultures, savoring diverse cuisines, and immersing ourselves in the beauty of the world without the booze. Sounds weird but I can now imagine traveling with a heightened sense of clarity and presence. I never had that. I know I missed so much while I was traveling because I was too wasted to take it in or too hungover I would waste the day away in my hotel room.

Sobriety will now allow us to fully absorb the richness of each travel experience, creating lasting memories and forging connections with people and places. I can't wait!

A future without Jungle Juice unfolds as a vibrant mosaic created with intention, purpose, and the transformative power of sobriety. Each brick represents a choice, a commitment to living authentically, and a step towards a life of fulfillment and well-being. As we embark on this sober life, visualize the possibilities that await. Remember how I said if you can imagine it, you can achieve it! Let the vision of a future without alcohol guide you towards a life rich in meaning, connection, and joy. It's there! Let's move through it, achieve it and enjoy it!

CHAPTER 20
Keep Growing and Going

How do we embrace clarity? What is clarity?

I have known clarity a couple of times in my life. Now is certainly one of them. I find that I have clarity when I have goals, motivation, drive, ambition to reach those goals. It's a sense of growth and change in your life. It's hard to explain. It's a feeling, like love is.

You may feel a more "spiritual connection" like I do. Obviously, I can't speak for you, but I have a feeling that you believe like I do that there is something bigger than us out there. Call it what you want but when you feel connected to that source things just feel better, clearer.

There's no distraction from your perseverance, like a bull in a china shop – you just GO!

You may be so completely clear in your life that you just have a take no bullshit presence and attitude, which may come off as cocky or people may label you as a bitch – it's not. They are entitled to their opinions. It's just confidence. It may even get to a point that you are so clear in your direction that you are leaving others behind as you learn, focus and grow. You may actually outgrow some people in your life.

That is okay… Just like every flower that blooms in a garden – it doesn't hold back, it doesn't wait for others it just has this innate confidence to just go and grow. If others catch up then that's amazing, they will stand tall and create a beautiful garden. If they don't, then they weren't strong enough and ready to grow. But if that one flower is the only one flower to bloom in the space it will be the most beautiful and get the most attention. I have learned that the only constant in life is change. Sometimes we need to change our circle because our circle doesn't change.

Being on this journey is such a ride, it's amazing how many ideas and opportunities arise when you have a clear mind to let new ideas and thoughts come in that will enable you to blast through life.

The journey of recovery from alcohol abuse is a profound and transformative one that extends beyond the mere cessation of substance use. It is a voyage of self-discovery, resilience, and continuous personal growth. In this chapter we're going to focus on yourself and your new life with new surroundings. I'm going to dive into the pivotal role played by mindfulness, self-reflection, and ongoing personal development in the journey of living authentically free.

I really want to focus on nurturing a holistic approach to healing, this idea aims to unravel the interconnected threads that weave together clarity, empowerment, and sustained sobriety. Don't worry – I'm not going to get all hippy dippy with you but I am going to encourage you to think beyond your current beliefs and to trust the process that you are going through even though it may feel like quick sand sometimes.

We have got to have a complete understanding of the foundations of clarity to enable us to thrive moving forward. I have compiled an incredible list to help you navigate your transformation.

Quitting booze isn't just about putting the bottle down. It's about so much more. The more you tap into self-discovery with the willingness to learn from yourself and others it will throw you in the trajectory to keep on keeping on.

Let's chat about a few key ideas to get us started. We always hear the big wig gurus and well, the wanna be big wigs talk about "mindfulness practice" or to practice "mindfulness." What the fuck does that even mean? Many of you are probably thinking… "All I fucking do is think. I don't want to anymore. This is why I drink because I'm done feeling and thinking."

I was the same way, but believe me when I say it's a necessary tool to work with to enable you to get through this.

So… What is mindfulness? Especially mindfulness in recovery?

Mindfulness, rooted in the practice of being fully present in the current moment, serves as the cornerstone of recovery from alcohol use and abuse. It offers a lens through which we can observe our thoughts, emotions, and behaviors without judgment. Mindfulness practices, such as meditation and deep-breathing exercises, become powerful tools in developing heightened self-awareness.

Being fully present, often associated with the concept of mindfulness, refers to the state of being completely engaged and attentive to the current moment, without distraction or preoccupation with the past or future. This is vitally important. Knowing when to let things go. We can't control or change the past and we literally have no idea what the future has in store for us, so what's the point of worrying about it? You are only one thought away from a decision that could change your life, forever!

This involves cultivating a heightened awareness of your thoughts, feelings, and the surrounding environment, fostering a deep connection with the present experience.

"Okay, I'm here, I'm alive, that means I'm 'present', right?"

Wrong.

Are you really present though?

Let me share some ideas on how we can change our own busy narrative to allow space for actually being "in the moment." It's more than just waking up and saying, "Okay, I'm here." Let's get deeper than that and unload what it really means.

1. Mindful Awareness: This means being fully present and it requires a conscious and intentional attention to the present moment. It involves observing thoughts, emotions, and sensations without judgment, allowing for a clear and non-reactive awareness.

Without judgment. I talked about this earlier. It's so fucking hard not to beat ourselves up for shit we did in the past. Trust me! I know the feeling. In all actuality, though, what is there that we can do about it? I'll tell you – FUCK ALL!

When you are starting to practice your mindfulness – yep, it's going to feel awkward and uncomfortable. You may only get 30 seconds in, but keep going every day and you will naturally invite more time in. When a negative thought comes to mind, literally tell it, "Thank you for sharing, I'm busy right now", and then get back to walking your dog and watching him sniff and piss on every leaf you walk by and give him a little scratch with a laugh and tell him how silly he is. This right here is mindfulness. If you are out with your dog, just be out with your dog. Other things can wait.

Keep full attention to the task at hand, whether it be walking your dog, planting your garden, mowing the lawn or having a one on one uninterrupted conversation with the person you are interacting with. When was the last time you actually listened to a friend without interjecting and talking about your past or you and you just focused on what they were saying? This focused attention enhances the quality of experiences, relationships, and activities by avoiding divided attention or multitasking. In interpersonal interactions, being fully present means giving undivided attention to others, especially your friends and family. Just like you expect and accept when they are there for you, make sure you are there for them back. We are all going through shit in our lives. You don't want to be that "all about me" person. Your friends are your friends for a reason and believe you me, it's not because you talk about yourself all the time. Just because you are going through your own personal struggles you mean and matter to somebody. Don't forget to engage with active listening, empathetic understanding, and genuine engagement in the conversation or shared experience with your gal pals and show them that they mean something to you too. Anyone, really. Just like you would expect undivided attention, it's fair to return it.

2. Acceptance of the Present: Well there you have it, you woke up today either feeling like a bag of shit or ready to face the day. This is all you've got. It's up to you and only you to be fully engaged in the present moment which involves accepting it as it is, right now, without resistance or the desire for it to be different. This acceptance allows for a more profound connection with the current circumstances. Don't worry if you don't want to hang out there for long. This too shall pass. Have solace in knowing that. Just like things aren't the exact same as they were a week ago they most certainly aren't going to be the same a week from now.

3. Emotional Presence: This is a tough one for me because I've often been called out for being soulless, especially with my resting bitch face. I remember so clearly in high school even teachers would tell me to smile when walking down the hall. When I was personal training, other staff would motion with their fingers to smile. Was I THAT dead inside, that soulless bitch is what I was putting out into the world? Yikes! I've been so guarded with my emotions that I have never really shared them with a spouse, friends, family. I would only share with myself through writing.

We all have emotions. We do. I'm still working on this to find mine and to stop being so tactful and by the book and orderly. I have a hard time with my femininity in a relationship (I've always been this way) because I am such an alpha. I grew up early and I grew up fast, that my childhood experiences have led me to a leadership role many times in my life. I'm unable to segregate those roles. As my dad would always say, "I is what I is and I ain't what I ain't."

But being fully present includes acknowledging and experiencing emotions in real-time. It involves not suppressing or avoiding emotions but rather allowing them to arise, be felt, and pass without attachment or judgment. "But I don't wanna," you say. I hear you! "I don't wanna" either. Stuffing all that shit down is terrible for us though. We gotta talk about it. Hence, this book. I've got shit to unload. It's been bogging me down. I need to make room for all the goodness in my life that I now expect and deserve. It's time to talk.

4. Sensory Awareness: Sounds kind of far out there but I mean this really makes sense (no pun intended) if you think about it – but we were given the 5 senses so that we could experience life on this earth. Let's utilize them. What if we started engaging our senses and took notice that they play a crucial role in being fully present. This involves noticing the sights, sounds, smells, tastes, and tactile sensations of the present moment, creating a richer and more immersive experience. If you are smelling the coffee now, you are here now in this moment, you are present. Smell it, enjoy it. If you fucking hate coffee think of another situation that your sense of smell is so overpowered that it hits you in the face? I bet that when you walk in your bathroom after your husband leaves and THAT smell almost knocks you over, you are definitely there in that moment and are present for it – it's alllll you can smell. Am I right or am I right? Now take that moment of *intensity* and apply it as you venture throughout your day. Pretending that everything smells like shit... Lol. You know what I mean! Be in those moments and fully present.

5. Absence of Distractions: Get rid of those distractions. The dishes will still be there when you get back. Like really they aren't going anywhere. Being fully present requires minimizing external and internal distractions. This could involve putting away your phone, quieting the mind, and creating an environment that fosters focused attention. Take a break when you need. I've started telling John if I'm getting overwhelmed in my day that "I need a timeout" or "I'm putting myself to bed." Just cuz we are all kewl and adult like now, doesn't mean that we aren't allowed to take a time out. It's necessary to take a step back, and just chill for a few minutes.

6. Timelessness: Have you ever experienced that when you are fully present, you may experience a sense of timelessness. It's sort of like the past and future lose their grip, and there is a profound sense of "now", where each moment unfolds without the weight of what has been or the anticipation of what's to come. It's okay if you haven't felt this before. Keep an eye open for it, it may just come up and surprise you and you will remember reading this, chuckle a little and say to yourself, "Challaine mentioned this might happen. She was right."

7. Increased Intuition and Creativity: This is what I was talking about earlier on in this chapter. That sense of connecting or that knowing of something greater out there, or just having a "feeling" about something – that right there is your intuition or your gut. When you have clarity in your mind it's like your intuition is supercharged and you literally are way more in tune with your "gut feeling." It's so much easier to tap into this when you are sober. You trust yourself more. When you are bogged down by booze, it's impossible to "trust your gut" cuz your gut doesn't even know what it wants. It's drunk too.

If your gut is drunk, your mind is drunk which in turn means you have zero clarity. Too many crossed wires to enable synchronicity and for your mind and body to work synergistically together.

When you are fully present you often tap into your intuition and creativity more readily. For me, I don't second guess myself as much. I trust myself more. The absence of mental clutter allows for fresh insights and a heightened ability to navigate challenges or generate innovative ideas. Since being sober the amount of brilliant ideas that I have come up with has been outstanding and exciting. I didn't even go out looking for these ideas. I released the poison from my mind which paved the way for the universe to send me the ideas and thoughts that will change my life – like this very book.

8. Reduced Stress and Anxiety: Don't you want to reduce your stress and decrease or eliminate your anxiety?

Spoiler alert. Get off the booze! "But I've had a stressful day, I need a drink." No, you don't. You've just conditioned yourself to believe that's what you need. Your mind may be mentally stressed from a stressful day at work, but if you add booze into the mix you are now adding a physical stressor and increasing the stress hormone called cortisol which has many negative effects, one of them being that it stores fat, especially in the mid section, which then gives you something more to stress out about. Some other side effects of too much cortisol include: rounding of the face, acne, thinning skin, easy bruising, flushed face, slow healing, muscle weakness, severe fatigue, irritability, difficulty concentrating, high blood pressure, and headaches.

Being fully present can contribute to a sense of calm and reduced stress. When the mind is focused on the current moment, worries about the future or regrets about the past are minimized, leading to a more peaceful state of mind.

Practicing mindfulness and cultivating the ability to be fully present is a skill that can be developed through various techniques such as meditation, deep breathing exercises, and conscious awareness practices. By embracing this state of being, you may find increased fulfillment, deeper connections, and a richer experience of life. I know I am. I'm on a fucking roll and theres no stopping me!

The how's on doing the above are coming right up in the next few chapters.

This is about to get heavy so go ahead, grab a bevy (funny how that term means something different to me now), maybe a journal to take notes (or not) and chill. We're going to play around a bit and dig deep.

CHAPTER 21

Evolution Of Personal Growth

Personal Growth

Continuous personal growth is the dynamic force propelling me forward in my recovery journey. It involves an ongoing commitment to learning, adapting, and evolving. I've said it before and I'll keep saying it. The only constant in this world is change. Have you noticed that when you are stuck in drinking patterns your whole fucking life is stuck?

Your weight is stuck or increasing, your friend circle is low vibration, doesn't change and isn't fulfilling anymore? You can't seem to make more money or keep the money you have. How can your life change if you don't change your life? Like seriously though. How can you expect different results if you continue to do the exact same thing every day? "Just calling a spade a spade" (one of John's favourite phrases) but here's the real answer.. It won't!

As we shed old beliefs, patterns and habits and embrace new perspectives, they pave the way for a future that aligns with our truest selves. Our authentic selves. The one that is really in there. Trust me, she's there. She may be scared, shy, guarded but she's fucking strong. Look at all the hard bullshit that has happened in your life that you have overcome and you made it through, because you are fucking badass. I bet you didn't get through everything you did, by yourself, did you? You had friends, family, your dog, your bird, prayer. Whatever… So why would you think you can get through this alone? Reading this book, you aren't alone. I'm with you. We all need a little help sometimes and that's okay! Embrace that.

Once we get rid of the garbage in our minds and in our physical lives it opens the path for new ideas, creativity, new beliefs about ourselves and others to come into your life. You begin to set boundaries for what bull shit you will put up with from yourself or with others.

The evolution of personal growth during alcohol recovery is a transformative journey marked by self-discovery, resilience, and ongoing development. As we navigate the challenges of overcoming alcohol dependence (this isn't me but many others), alcohol addiction or alcohol habit (this is me) we embark on a path of profound change and self-improvement. Following is an idea of the evolution of personal growth throughout alcohol recovery and your journey to living authentically free. You may find yourself in one of these, or maybe a few. Nothing is ever set in stone so you can use this as a guideline or a bible. Whatever works for you. Be flexible with yourself, your emotions and your journey. We all learn and grow at a different pace. Just like children.

Acknowledgment and Acceptance

Recognition of the Problem
Such an icky word. No one, and I mean NO one likes to say, "I have a drinking problem." Maybe it's more along the lines of "Yeah, it's getting a little much" or "Yeah, I can tone it down" or "I don't HAVE to drink tomorrow." Why do we have to use the word "problem"? Why do we want to feel shitty about something that is already making us feel shitty? Let's change the narrative with our recognition towards the use of alcohol instead? Like "This isn't working for me anymore. Things gotta change" or "I don't really want to wake up feeling like this anymore." I don't know about you, but I have never said and never plan on saying "I have a problem with alcohol." It just puts me down and makes me feel like a shitty human. We need

to make ourselves feel good and lift ourselves up. Getting sober is fucking awesome! It's NOT a problem!

It's interesting how a few words can make all the difference. This initial step simply involves recognizing the impact of alcohol on your life, well-being, health, family, friends, work, etc and paving the way for self-awareness to do better. Instead of "I have a problem with alcohol", we can say "I have a solution to my problem with alcohol." That just FEELS inspiring.

Acceptance of the Need for Change
Once you have accepted that you are not going to live that life anymore, you have got to acknowledge what needs to change, and accept it. The recognition and understanding that change is necessary is vital to your recovery. You can realistically live any life you can imagine for yourself but NOT in your current state, otherwise you would be on that path to living that life right now. Well, isn't that a *Brain Wow* moment? Once you have the realization that alcohol is hindering your personal growth and commit to embracing a different, healthier lifestyle step by step and working on it daily – you can achieve greatness!

Early Stages of Sobriety

Detoxification and Physical Healing
The early stages of abstaining from jungle juice is terrible. Maybe you have tried getting sober before, make it a day or two and then relapse because the withdrawal is disgusting. Realistically, why would you want to put yourself through that when you can just avoid the whole thing by continuing doing what you have been doing? I think we revert back to drinking because we just aren't actually ready to get sober. Soulfully ready.

I'm telling ya, if you can get past what your body is saying to you with the pain of withdrawal and begin to listen to what you know to be true in your mind about alcohol and your life then you have a greater chance of success. You need one more step though. It's Body, Mind, *Soul*... All 3 need to work synergistically together for you to become free.

I'm gonna be blunt with you here. The only way to live an authentically free life free from booze is through it. You can't walk around it, you can't talk your way out of it – you literally just have to go through the motions and as they say "one step at a time." I would like to add to that, "one thought at a time."

At the beginning the steps are like the long jump in the Olympics, but as each day passes your long jumps turn into walks and then skips because you are so freaking excited that you are making it through and you know you can do it. You are starting to get some clarity as the poison is leaving your brain and body.

This is an amazing process that the body goes through. It want's to be there for you, support you but it needs to rest for a little bit. Give it that rest. As the toxicity is leaving your body and you feel like absolute shit, love it, thank it for the fun times and the drunken adventures you've had together but it's friendship is no longer needed. It's served its purpose to teach you all the many life lessons you have come to learn and realize and you are letting it go.

You only welcome health, vitality, and authenticism.

It's tough and you want to cave cuz you know what will make you feel better – a little "hair of the dog" is what I call it (aka – a drink). I urge you not to. It's only "fun" in the moment. We want to think about our goals and have the end goal in mind. If you cave – you already know what you are doing tomorrow – absolutely nothing because that one drink is going to lead to more and you just continue the cycle. You go from being hungover to just drunk again. Habits only break if you break the habits. No wonder it's so fucking hard because it's a HABIT! Imagine just not brushing your teeth when you normally do? Super weird right? Of course it is, because it is a habit!

21. Evolution Of Personal Growth

Physical healing is a crucial aspect of personal growth during this period, setting the stage for a healthier foundation. Give yourself some grace here!

Building a Support System

Establishing a strong support system becomes pivotal. Connecting with others who understand the challenges of recovery provides encouragement, empathy, and a sense of community, fostering early personal growth.

Easier said than done, right? Your support system is probably the people who you have been drinking with albeit friends, family or even co-workers. Everyone who knows "you." There's a weird sense of them judging you for "having a problem", there's a weird sense of your friendship changing. I have friends who's relationship with me is built on booze use and abuse. Every single time we got together we would just drink and I mean DRINK!

Part of you feels this unexplainable "weakness" in a sense, succumbing to the fact that you are unable to handle it anymore.

This can be freaking tough, but let me tell you… There is absolutely nothing weak about giving something up that has controlled your emotions, your finances, your health, your relationships – essentially your whole life.

Do you know how powerful you are to be able to set your own personal boundaries for what you will allow in your life?

What do these boundaries look like for you?

I don't necessarily have any that are too outlandish to be honest – but that is just me. You may have some strong and thick boundaries as your journey with booze may have been deeper than mine.

For me…

I don't give a flying fuck if people drink around me. I'm strong enough in my own skin and my own soul that I won't be tempted anymore. I'm just so over it.

I will find fun, safe and healthy alternatives when it comes to what I'm drinking and my environment. I promise not to judge others for doing what they want with their bodies as I expect the same in return...

I do expect those I hang out with to respect the fact that I'm not drinking anymore and not be like, "Oh, come on, it's just one", but I also expect that I still be included in events even though I'm not drinking anymore. Our friendships couldn't have only been based around alcohol, could they?

To be honest, they could.

I am open to maintaining the friendships I have had while being a drunk ass but are they comfortable hanging out with me because they want to drink and I don't? I'm sure you have said it to sober people around you, "Just have one drink with me." Misery loves company and when there's people around, you like to drink with them. You feel kind of dumb drinking by yourself in front of them. It's just a thing.

It's a tough reality but you may lose some friends in the process. It's going to be because of them though, not you. Remember that! You absolutely cannot blame your loss of friendship on your choice to get healthy. Maybe read that again. That's all you are doing...getting healthy. If you lose friends over that then I don't think you need those people anyways.

If someone doesn't want to hang out with you anymore because you are no longer drinking buddies that's okay. Look at it this way, though... If someone doesn't want to socialize with you anymore because you are getting healthy, fit, strong, clear minded, determined, goal oriented, all it does is say a LOT about them and volumes about you. For me, I've committed to not drinking and that's where I'm at right now. What others put in their bodies is none of my business, but I will and I am setting boundaries with my people and environment.

Go, go out and find new friends! I am! Why not? Look back in your life and look at all of the friends who have come and gone. Everyone who has come into your life at one point

21. Evolution Of Personal Growth

or another serves a purpose as a teacher or a student. There is always something to be learned from every relationship you are in – with your parents, friends, partners, – whomever.

If the relationship doesn't serve YOU anymore, it's okay to let it dissolve.

With social media there's an insane amount of support groups. You can just sit back and idly watch the reels as they go by about people's addictions and recovery. You can actively participate and ask questions or you may even surprise yourself and be able to offer some support ex: it's "only" been 1 day for someone trying to get sober, and they feel like they can't keep going (in more ways than one) – and you are "only" 5 days in but you share with them how you are climbing out of your 5th day, how it still hurts but you did it. Just that little bit of motivation could change or save someone's life. You are more powerful than you think.

At the end of the day, though, having a support system is important but there's nothing more important than being your own best friend! Be your own support system first, be your own friend to be there for you. Start doing what you love. As we know for me, it was writing! I'm finally writing my damn book! No wonder it's taken me almost a decade to write it. Have you ever tried reading while drinking? Impossible, well… writing while drinking, next level not happening.

Be there for yourself and let your light shine and you will be amazed at who ventures into your life.

What happens to dandelions in the morning when the sun comes out? They reach for it? Be the sun in your own world and watch the friendship flowers bloom all around you.

At the end of the day, everyone goes to bed in their own bodies and their own minds, as great as it is to have others, know in your heart that you have YOU, first and foremost.

Navigating Challenges and Resilience

Confronting Triggers

Personal growth unfolds as you confront and navigate triggers associated with alcohol.

But the fucking triggers, they are everywhere! Social media, magazines, tv commercials, restaurants, strip malls. How do we get past them?

You don't! Plain and simple… So again, switch the narrative. They quite honestly just can not and will not be your triggers anymore. Commit.

For the most part these triggers are paid advertisements to get you to drink their product, and guess what? The more you drink their product, the more you will drink their product. It's like marketing genius or something.

Actually, it's more like brainwashing. It's false advertising in a sense.

Prescription drug companies list all the side effects of their medications. If alcohol is a drug then why don't they list or advertise theirs? You never see the aftermath after a night of drinking or the morning after the night before on the tv ads. The fights, the yelling, the stripping, the puking, the cops, the hangovers.

All they are required to say is "Drink Responsibly." Is that even a thing? How the fuck do you drink responsibly? Maybe I can't personally identify with it as I described in my previous chapter because I was never able to do it.

Have you noticed people on your Facebook taking selfies with their alcoholic bevy in their hand? Why is this a thing? Look at that sneaky alco elf – just creeping in there and photo-bombing your pics.

Selfies are generally for #1 – yourself or #2 – you and your friends. Not you and booze. It's so ridiculous to me now "Look at me, getting wasted and losing all self control."

I USED to look at others' pics and see that and think, "They are having so much fun" but now I look and I see red skin, puffy eyes, exhaustion, unhealthy bodies. Keeping in mind a lot of my circle are nineties girls too and I can promise you that they didn't just start drinking yesteryear. The booze is catching up with them now too.

Developing resilience and resistance in the face of these everyday challenges becomes a hallmark of ongoing development. Trust me, no need for FOMO here. You KNOW what happens after a night of drinking. You don't want to go there anymore, it's not a fun place to be.

Learning Healthy Coping Mechanisms

Our evolution through our alcoholic behaviors involves replacing maladaptive coping mechanisms or habits with healthy alternatives. Learning constructive ways to manage stress, anxiety, time and emotions is a crucial step in this.

Mid-Recovery and Establishing Foundations
Let's talk about self-discovery.

So you are traversing through or you have made it across to the other side of the acceptance and mandatory shitty withdrawal process. Where does that leave you now?

Let's call it something like mid-recovery? This could come quickly for you, like speedy fast or it could take time to rear its head. For me it was FAST. Like I was on a timeline and had shit to do – NOW! This marks a period of self-discovery where you are so motivated that you can take on the world.

This is where people get serious about their values, interests, and aspirations, rediscovering aspects of themselves that may have been overshadowed by alcohol use. It's such a cool thing to pop up. It's like an unexpected but welcomed slap in the face.

Establishing Routine and Structure
My daily routines and habits consisted of grabbing a bottle at about 3pm so I would have a nice glow on before the big kids

got home by 4:15 or so. That would give me enough time to get some supper started, start my third glass of wine and have at least three smokes. As we know, my glasses were always spritzed, so not as much wine as one would think, although as the glass would go down I would top up with wine so the spritz would be less and less as the night went on. I wine'd my spritz, not spritzed my wine.

I would feel alive and accomplished knowing I was creating a masterpiece in the kitchen for my humans.

I would be excited to see them walk in the door as I was whipping up some amazing food for them. But, I was also counting down the minutes before they walked in, so I could get one last smoke in my lungs. They hate my smoking. No kidding. I was definitely at times a smoke sneaker. Let's be honest, though, it smells so bad that there's nothing sneaky about it.

I'm living in my brand new million dollar house, drinking out of my fine crystal wine glasses. What could be wrong with that? That's what all the rich moms do on tv. They've got their shit together. Millions in the bank, successful businesses and just loved their wine. No harm done.

Wrong.

In the moment, it was all fine and dandy. I had energy, creativity, a smile on my face, but…

I was at the point where I wouldn't put my babies to bed until 9-10 o'clock at night cuz I wanted to "hang out with them" but in hindsight I didn't want to be away from my glass for the half hour that it would take to change them, read them a book and put them to bed. You know how much drinking can get done in that time frame? Like I said, almost three glasses and at least three smokes.

I was in my happy spot as I was watching "my show" on Netflix. I've never been a Netflix and chill kinda girl. It's always Netflix and cook. I would plan out my cooking, in line with my drinking so that one step would be done, I could fill up then take five to go smoke and drink my wine.

21. Evolution Of Personal Growth

But the aftermath was everything short of enjoyable. The afternoons turned into nightly routines of cooking with the wine glass in my hand which led to the same routine every morning of being hungover. It didn't matter if I had a Tylenol, Alka Seltzer, water and electrolytes before bed. The mornings still consisted of one or all of the following: headaches, grogginess, having the shits, no appetite, anxiety, being exhausted, no motivation, no drive, denial that I was hungover. "I'm just tired" was my catchphrase. No shit I was "just tired." My body just ran a marathon while drinking ethanol!

Scrap energy, creativity and a smile on my face. I dreaded getting out of bed – some days I just wouldn't cuz I couldn't. Like I actually couldn't physically move.

Call it luck, sure. I guess I was extremely lucky that I HAD to go to work 14 hours away from my house. To detox in a hotel room, lie in my own self-pity and shitty thoughts and just feel defeated. Who knows where I would be if I had stayed at home. Leaving my children is always so hard for me but if I didn't then I wouldn't be where I am today.

If you don't change your circumstances or your environment then your circumstances and environment won't change. Easy concept, right? Sure. We are creatures of habit. I had to go.

The bigs will always have the memory of me being dragged out of my house in my booty shorts and spaghetti strap tank top, shoeless, handcuffed and put in the back of a cop car, being absolutely belligerent to the officers. This was the night I assaulted my ex.

Before I left for work at the beginning of January, PaLoma, my oldest daughter saw me stumbling in the bathroom cuz I was so wasted. She will remember that forever just like I remember my mother falling in the middle of the night hammered trying to get the washroom at my Godparents house.

I'm sorry, you two. That is never a way to see your mother.

What I do want you to see is that habits can be broken. That if you commit to something and want to get shit done you will do it! I'm sorry it took me so long to get to this point, but I did and I couldn't be prouder of myself. I hope you are proud of me too. Fighting that beast was a fucking challenge.

What does this mean for me going home after being on the road for a month?

Lots!

I've always been an all or nothing kinda girl, and that's why I could never have "just one." When I get home I will be clear minded, setting different routines and schedules. Embracing new patterns and habits. Being fully present. Not being separated from my children with a crystal filter.

If you are struggling with the continual habit of alcohol use. Get away! Get away from your environment. Go to a hotel to detox, go stay with your parents, go to an actual rehab facility, go to a friend's house and stay in the guest room for four days. Do whatever you need to do to break the habit. The routine was the problem for me.

Time and place can change people. Give yourself the time to get the alcohol out of your system and start over. I'm living proof that it's possible.

Our personal growth is facilitated by the establishment of an implemented routine and structure. Implementing a daily schedule and engaging in positive habits can and will contribute to stability, a new drive to get up every day and a sense of purpose.

Embracing Therapeutic Interventions

Engaging in Therapy

Personal growth can deepen through therapeutic interventions. I'm no stranger to therapy. I started at an early age. I strongly believe that everyone can benefit from therapy. What's the harm in getting all of the shit that is inside of you, out? Our emotions bottled up can manifest into physical turbulence such as anxiety. With the anxiety from drinking mixed with the anxiety from bottled up emotions can be absolutely crippling.

21. Evolution Of Personal Growth

Coincidental for me? I think not... My physical anxiety manifested within my throat. I believe for more reasons than one. But here's my first one... I have a huge fear about choking. This stems from when I was young and it was the holidays. I was with my mother and she ended up choking on a turkey vertebra of all things, believe it or not. The ambulance ended up coming and taking her to the hospital. Another time my mother choked I had to give her abdominal thrusts behind her, she then ended up on the floor and I had to essentially keep giving her compressions to dislodge the blockage.

To this day, I am still terrified of choking. I've had to literally pull food out of JorDhyn and LunDhyn's throats as I knew in an instant they were choking. JorDhyn was with a fry and Lunny with a strawberry.

I also have really bizarre eating habits. John can eat three burgers and a large fry (no lie) and I still won't be finished with a small order of fries. I chew my food to an absolute mush. I cannot carry a conversation while I'm eating. Anxiety goes through the roof.

I have to leave the room if I'm around my mother and she is eating. Unfortunately, I'm still at a point where I'm unable to have holiday dinners with her. I will bring her food but I can't be around when she eats.

I remember the first time I had trouble swallowing. I was coming home from the gym and I had drank a whole N.O.S. energy drink and was driving. I had to pull over midway home because my heart was racing and I couldn't even swallow my own saliva.

Ever since that time I have had issues with my throat. The excess caffeine had "activated" a physical trauma response in my body where my throat just couldn't operate the way it needed to.

Drinking alcohol would make it go away but then the next day it would come back with a vengeance. My hangovers would be so bad I could only sip on water to wet my lips. I couldn't chug the water that my body so desperately needed.

It got so bad that I explained to my doctor what was going on and she sent me for a swallowing test. Yep! It's a thing. It's actually called an esophagogram or a "barium swallow." The test is designed to test the upper gastrointestinal tract for GERD (gastrointestinal reflux disease), hiatal hernias, ulcers and tumors. Candidates for this test include those who have abdominal pain, bloating, vomiting and you guessed it... trouble swallowing.

So... I did the test and – surprise, surprise – I was perfectly healthy in my upper GI tract.

If everything was okay with me physically from what they could see based on the test, then the only other palpable answers to my difficulty swallowing is my past traumas with my mother in regards to swallowing, my own personal experience with difficulties swallowing from increased caffeine or the fact that I may have Dysphagia.

Dysphagia is a condition which is where a person has trouble swallowing and prolonged alcohol use can be a contributing factor. Prolonged alcohol abuse can lead to malnutrition which in turn can affect the brain to body response in the esophageal muscles. Any proper muscular function to be precise. Alcohol is significant in the depletion of B vitamins in the body. As a reminder, B vitamins are essential for cellular and metabolic functioning. They are also water soluble which means that they are dissolved in water and since alcohol depletes and dehydrates us of H2O it takes the B vitamins out with the trash. Add the fact that we most likely aren't eating the correct foods when we are constantly consuming alcohol, we aren't replenishing our vitamin B stores, which should be done daily. Vitamin B is responsible for so many functions in our body including brain function, cell health, proper nerve function and digestion to name a few. If you look at any medical journal it is mentioned that digestion begins in the mouth.

Let me pull this all in for you. Layman's terms....

Vitamin B deficient= nerve, brain and digestion dysfunction= trouble swallowing. Now I'm no doctor but I'm going to suggest that my drinking in conjunction with my choking traumas and lack of proper nutrition have completely disabled the neural pathways to function properly. So for me this is a two-step process for recovery for this. Continue to see my therapist about my choking traumas that began with my mother and increase my B vitamins.

Count me in.

By engaging in individual or group therapy it allows us to explore underlying issues, gain insights, and develop strategies for long-term recovery. It's so important to get all that's in you, out.

Advanced Recovery and Sustaining Progress

Pursuing Educational and Career Goals

Are you stuck in your life? Are you not feeling fulfilled in your soul? Have you lost your connection to yourself? If you haven't then I would be incredibly surprised.

Not only does alcohol affect us physically it takes away our minds, goals and dreams.

I have always been a serial learner. A student for life and a student of life.

I talked earlier about all of the courses that I was signed up for and didn't complete. There is seriously no reason why these courses didn't get completed other than the fact I spent my time drinking instead of studying, then I would lose interest and just not continue the courses at all.

Does this sound familiar?

My goals were all over the place and I didn't take any action in order to reach those goals. Okay, maybe not "any action" but certainly not the action needed to propel me forward in the trajectory of my accomplished goals. So essentially I just had wishes.

NOW... Now that I'm sober I have such a clear vision of where I want my life to go. The action steps that I need to take in order to get there and I have such a physical and mental knowing, without any question that I will accomplish what I set out to do. Provided, it may not be on the timeline I want but it is going to happen. It is happening.

In three months I have curated and created this book. How? Because I stepped away from the bottle and into my mind but most importantly my soul. I have established a universal connection with all that is creative, divine and all knowing in itself. I have developed a trust – a trust in the process but most importantly a trust in myself that alcohol took away.

Not only have the relationships in my life changed for the good, the relationship with myself has changed drastically. I am so much more connected to who I am in my soul. By my soul, I mean the inner me that makes me feel, love, know and trust. The soul that is connected to nature and the eternal creator or source.

When you can learn to surrender and just trust and know without a doubt that everything is okay in the end and that if it's not okay, then it's not the end. Life just flows like a river, merrily down the stream. It's not forced anymore like a river trying to flow up the stream.

Continuous Self-Improvement.
Now I'm not saying that I have found the be all and end all. Fuck no!

This is a process and it will continue to be a process for the rest of my life.

I will still need to process temptation, process doubt, process and work through failure, process all of my lessons learned. The alcohol and the problems that it hosts may be gone but it doesn't change the fact that life will always be full of challenges and its own hurdles that I will move through.

Being unchained from the grips of alcohol enables us to deal with these obstacles as mole hills, not mountains. We develop the mental resilience to better understand our surroundings, other people, and, most importantly, ourselves.

We continue to grow in a direction with less tension, more love, understanding and compassion for self and others.

In order to do this we can't think of sobriety as linear.

Personal growth in alcohol recovery is an ongoing process with ups and downs. Engaging in continuous learning, seeking opportunities for self-improvement through workshops, courses, and the pursuit of new skills will begin to align your SMART goals. These are Specific, Measurable, Achievable, Relevant and Time Sensitive. Write them down. What are your goals? Get SMART with them.

Resilience in the Face of Setbacks

Now I know this is awe inspiring and it's exciting seeing your future blossom ahead of you, although I don't sugar coat anything. You will continue to face failures and obstacles. I want you to know that relapses or challenges can be a part of the recovery journey. They aren't stop signs! As each day goes by and you are so dead set focused on your sobriety, relationships and real self-authenticity you will continue to learn and grow. Remember we talked earlier about the lesson will continue to be taught until it is learned?

Mentoring and Giving Back

Supporting Others in Recovery

We are certainly better together.

People are meant to people together. We are meant for community, connection and family.

Now I get it. Every family dynamic is different and what "family" is to me may not be the same for you. That's totally fine. If your family isn't by blood then so be it. Tori is my best friend on this planet, although she isn't blood related she is my sister from another mister. We have a relationship that is worth curating and working on and constantly developing.

Who's in your family? Don't have anyone?

GO GET SOMEONE! Go to your meetings, find your support groups, go meet your people. They are out there. I promise. They were meant for you. What you may have not realized though is that you are meant for them too.

A great way to meet people and to feel a sense of purpose is to volunteer. What activities or hobbies do you like or have? Love puppies? Go down to your local shelter and offer to volunteer. Guaranteed you will meet other people who love puppies there.

Do you like helping people? There's many opportunities for volunteers at hospitals or hospice centers. Consider the impact you would have on someone who is sick or in the process of their ultimate transition while being by themselves. To share stories, to feel compassion, to feel heard and to be seen. You can be that person for someone else.

What an act of love and service it is to help. When you can be of service to others, not only are you helping someone (which I believe is so important to help and serve where we can) you end up showing love to that person in need. They will feel cared for, important, worthy and loved just by you showing up. If you can make someone feel all of those things, there's only one plausible way that's possible.

Because you ARE all of those things.

Now isn't that beautiful?

Sometimes we enter each other's lives to be the teacher and/or the student while simultaneously to give and to receive love. What a gift!

Who can you be there for? I believe that you have the capacity within you, to be someone else's person. When I went to all of my women's sessions after the assault, I, like many, sat in that group and just listened, but once I started sharing my story, others started listening and we would have such in depth conversations and I was told, "Thank you for sharing" or "OMG, me too." When you share and communicate, not only can it be cathartic for you it can immeasurably help others without you even knowing. You will gain your own cheer squad and become someone else's cheer squad.

Talking and sharing can be scary. I get it. We are so wrapped in "I'm tough" to "I don't need anyone." Let me remind you of something. You were given a mouth with a voice for a reason and that reason is NOT to keep quiet. Share your story, share your life, share your heart. THAT'S how you find your people.

You were also given ears for listening. Relationships are about give and take. Personal growth extends by supporting others in their recovery journeys also. Those further along in their recovery often become mentors, providing guidance, empathy, and encouragement to individuals at earlier stages.

Where are you in your stage?

If you feel like this would never be you, where people don't care? Remember this… Don't think about the group of people who don't give a shit, think about that ONE person who does give a shit. You are speaking to THAT person.

Think back on your life. Is there one person who stands out for you that had such a profound impact on you? They motivated you, they inspired you, they changed you? How freakin' amazing do you feel just even thinking about that person? What gifts has that person provided for you emotionally or spiritually?

Now, what a gift of self-love to be able to offer your gifts of emotional or spiritual support to someone else.

You have it in you to be a secret gift giver – now how cool is that?

How can you share your gifts with the world?

Go Give & Take

CHAPTER 22
Mindful Path To Recovery

Before we can begin being mindful we need to have an understanding of what true mindfulness is. My interpretation is to have a deep and profound knowing that we are not as we see ourselves in the mirror. We are not human beings having a spiritual experience, we are spiritual beings having a human experience.

I want you to sit with that for a minute. We are spiritual beings having a human experience.

We talked about values earlier on. Our values, our beliefs, our intuition, our love. What is that? Where does it come from?

I believe that it comes from somewhere outside of our physical bodies. It comes from the universe, from the source, from the creator. So if it comes from that then it must without a doubt *be* that. If it comes from that and is in us, then we MUST also without a doubt, *be* that!

Okay, now talk about a *Brain Wow* moment right there.

When we can truly connect to, or be mindful of our core beliefs, ideas, values and love then we are connecting to the source that we came from. Pure perfection. A source that doesn't make mistakes, a source that has created everything in divine order to operate exactly as it should.

In case you didn't pick up what I'm saying: You are absolutely perfect!

I encourage you to tap into that perfection.

I know what you must be thinking. "How can I be perfect? I cheated, I stole, I lied", etc...

Those are things you DID not WHO you ARE. Big difference!

I also know that all of those things have happened to teach you a lesson, to enable you to be better. You may have not seen it in that particular moment but you did down the road.

Like when I was a serial cheater. It took me losing one of my greatest loves to realize that I couldn't do that to people anymore. It physically, emotionally and spiritually changed me. My lesson was learned. In my relationship with John I have been 100% faithful and don't have one ounce of regret or shame knowing that I betrayed him. That those old patterns and feelings are no longer a part of my being.

That's what this whole show called life is about, being taught the lesson until it is learned. This cultivates transformation so that the soul, the inner you can grow, love and connect to oneself – which if you are following along, will take you full circle back to the source.

Woah.

So how do we do this? It sounds like hogwash.

I've curated some ideas for you to help you to connect to yourself. Your inner self, to strengthen your beliefs, deepen your love for yourself and others and to gain a better perspective of how to navigate this life with compassion, resilience, truth, understanding and fortitude.

Cultivating Mindfulness Practices

Mindfulness practices, such as meditation and mindful breathing, offer practical spiritual and physical techniques for us to navigate the challenges of recovery. These practices provide a sanctuary for self-reflection, allowing us to observe cravings, emotions, relationships, and stressors with a non-judgmental awareness.

Cultivating mindfulness practices can be a valuable and transformative aspect of your journey to recovery from alcohol.

22. Mindful Path To Recovery

Mindfulness involves being fully present in the current moment. I know it's easier said than done.

This is not a one-time gig, though. It is a PRACTICE and must be practiced in order to master.

I always thought that I would be hit with this massive gut punch of a feeling when it came to meditation. That there would be some sort of immediate and major transformation. That's not what meditation is about. It is a journey of transformation where in time you will discover that your life and connections just flow so much easier and you are able to handle life with grace and ease. This is the ultimate goal of mindfulness practices.

Mindful practices will enable you to observe your thoughts and emotions without judgment. Here are some practical ways to incorporate mindfulness into your recovery process:

1. Mindful Breathing

Practice conscious and deliberate breathing exercises. Focus on the sensation of your breath as you inhale and exhale. This simple yet powerful practice helps anchor you to the present moment and can be done anytime, anywhere. It helps regulate your breath, heart rate and thoughts by activating a relaxation response in the body.

Set a timer... start with five minutes. In for four seconds, hold for four, out for seven.

In through your nose and expand your belly here, not your chest. Big difference. We want the breath in for four seconds to move life through you not just into you, hold for four seconds then exhale through your mouth for seven seconds. I want you to focus on the air leaving your entire body and releasing all of the shit – not just releasing air from your lungs. Sink into your out breath. Let your body fall by scanning your body, feeling each muscle release. Your jaw, your shoulders, your belly, your hips and all the way down. Systematically bring awareness to each part of your body. Notice any tension or sensations within and let them go, without judgment. This practice enhances body awareness and helps release physical and emotional stress.

2. Mindful Walking

I know that this can be a challenge for some people. To physically get up and leave the house. I know what you are thinking. You want me to go for a walk when showering or even brushing my teeth seems like a chore.

Yes! Yes, I do. I want you to get out of your house. There is literally no prerequisite to going for a walk. Nevermind the shower, nevermind brushing your teeth, just GO.

Maybe just going around the block is enough for day one. Make it two blocks the next day. Start with little goals. Set a timer and commit to 20 minutes, or 5,000 steps. Setting SMART goals will only encourage you to continue to set goals which are perfectly attainable. Maybe down the road you can invite someone to go with you, or maybe you want someone right off the hop? Get a dog and take him for a walk. I always meet people when I'm walking my dog.

I have yet to meet someone that has gone for a walk then said, "I really hated that I got some exercise and got to connect with nature while walking my dog today."

I get it, we don't like to be left with our own thoughts sometimes. That's totally fine. Listen to an audio book or podcast. Mel Robbins is absolutely incredible and has curated her podcasts to enable her listeners to move forward with strength, knowledge and resilience.

Dr. Wayne Dyer has been absolutely instrumental in my recovery. I have many of his books and his audio books. I've even got John listening to them when we are driving on the road. He recently said to me, "Did you ever think that you would be listening to Wayne Dyer with your husband while driving through the mountains?"

Honestly? No!

Mel Robbins and Wayne Dyer have been pillars in my life and have definitely helped me through my life's journey thus far and have been with me for many wins and losses over the past decade. I'm incredibly grateful for their wisdom.

4. Mindful Eating:

This doesn't start at the table. It starts before you even get to the grocery store. What can we eat to help repair our bodies after drinking and to begin living a sober lifestyle? How can we set ourselves up for success? I love me, a good old list.

What do you enjoy? How can we make that healthier? Do you eat Doritos everyday? Try some organic corn chips with an organic salsa for a change.

Little shifts in our nutrition can be hugely impactful when trying to incorporate a healthy diet. They can help to reduce sugar cravings (which also come in the form of starchy carbohydrates). We get addicted to these. Breads, pastas, rice, potatoes.

A great place to start is with nuts, seeds, berries, lean proteins like fish and turkey, while also incorporating plenty of other fruits and vegetables.

I am going to note here that I definitely don't recommend going to the grocery store while you are hungry. That's a terrible idea. Not only do we have the physical distraction of the hunger pangs and the lowered blood sugar but we have the mental battle of guilt and shame of actually putting the items in the cart. These feelings are then delivered to us again when we eat the unhealthy food and AGAIN after we eat it. That seems like a lot of stress for a box of cookies.

I also recommend eating every three hours so that the blood sugar doesn't dip so low that you need a quick fix so you end up hitting the drive through or going for that box of cookies (we know you're not having just one). More guilt, more shame.

Water is also vitally important. Keep a water bottle with you. Always. Set a timer to remind you to drink water if you need. Drinking water throughout the day can help keep the hunger pangs down and the sugar cravings low.

Practice mindful eating by savoring each bite of your meals. Pay attention to the taste, texture, and aroma of the food. Eating mindfully can enhance your appreciation for nourishing your body and prevent impulsive behaviors.

You've got this!

5. Guided Mindfulness Meditation:

A guided meditation is where someone literally guides you with their voice through the process on how to get into a meditative state.

We have this idea that we need to lie in Shavasana at the end of a yoga class to experience a guided meditation. However, we can literally meditate anywhere. I love to listen to guided meditations as I'm going to sleep curled up in a ball. There are numerous resources available, including apps, podcasts, audio books and online videos. There are also offerings of guided meditations specifically designed for addiction recovery.

It's not a one size fits all category. I've definitely listened to meditations where the person's voice wasn't a good fit for me. I actually prefer to listen to a man rather than a woman. I find that a deeper and calm tone resonates better with me for relaxation. *Headspace* and *Calm* are some great apps that provide accessible tools for integrating meditation into your life. YouTube also has an extensive library for meditation content.

6. Mindful Journaling

Now being an author, writing comes so naturally for me. I've been writing since I was in kindergarten. Journaling, actually. How are you with writing? Do the words just flow through you or is it a struggle? What do you write about?

Writing is a form of release and of self expression.

I definitely encourage you to write down your feelings as well as your gratefuls. It doesn't have to be long and elaborate. When you first start out it may or may not be so detailed but just get it out.

It could look like any of the following:

22. Mindful Path To Recovery

"I'm so grateful today that I haven't had a drink in a week. I'm really craving one though. The weather sucks and I wanted to go for a walk cuz it helps to clear my head but it's raining and really cold today. I'm grateful I woke up today, not hungover. I will try again tomorrow for the walk."

That's it, that's all. Simple. You were able to get some feelings out and got two gratefuls in. Practicing mindful gratitude by regularly reflecting on the positive aspects of your life, this can shift your focus away from perceived deficiencies and reinforce a positive mindset.

That's a WIN in my journal.

As with anything you want to get good at, you must practice. Writing is a skill that can be developed and so is sharing your soul. We bottle so much in, it can feel weird or even stupid to write or talk about it. That's okay to feel weird. Just keep going. Embrace being weird. Weird isn't a bad thing!

Incorporate mindful journaling into your routine, even if it's just a sentence or two a day. Just write!

Reflect on your thoughts, feelings, and experiences related to your past, your relationships and your recovery journey. This self-reflection can provide valuable insights and serve as a tool for tracking progress. I mean who doesn't like to reflect on the progress they have made?

I certainly do… It just makes me want to go for more!

Journaling is such a transformative tool for self-reflection. Through the written word, we release our thoughts, emotions, and progress, creating a tangible record of our journey and lives. Journaling serves as a mirror, reflecting the evolution of our mindset and fostering a deeper connection within ourselves.

Are you ready to go all in? Then freaking' do it!

A. Go Select Your Journal

There's nothing more satisfying than staring at the wall of beautiful journals at the bookstore, then picking them up, seeing the colours, the inspirational text on the cover or throughout while flipping through and smelling the blank crisp fresh pages.

Choose a journal that resonates with you though. It can be a simple notebook, a dedicated recovery journal, or even a digital journaling app if you prefer typing. Tip* Don't think too hard about this. The journal usually chooses you!

B. Set a Regular Time.

Establish a consistent time for journaling. Whether it's in the morning, during a quiet moment in the afternoon, or before bedtime. Having a regular time makes it easier to incorporate into your routine. I've got four children, so I definitely understand how busy you can be. There's absolutely no way in hell I would be able to "take five" during the day to get my practice done, so I have to create the time by getting up earlier than everyone in my house. My wake up time is 4am. That's when I get my writing in.

C. Create a Comfortable Space

Find a quiet and comfortable space to write. This can be a corner in your home, a park bench, or any place where you feel at ease and focused.

Reflect on your day then move into gratitude while exploring your emotions.

Don't know what to write? Start with facts. Actual facts. Reflect on your day, then consider your emotions, experiences, and any challenges you faced. Acknowledge both positive and challenging moments.

Write down a few things you are grateful for. Cultivating a gratitude practice can shift your focus towards the positive aspects of your life, promoting a more optimistic outlook.

Don't be shy to dive into your emotions. Don't worry about being raw and vulnerable. Nobody is going

22. Mindful Path To Recovery

to read it. It's just you. You can be honest with yourself. Remember the old saying "the truth shall set you free"?

Practice this here. You don't need to go into the nitty gritty right away about your deepest and darkest secrets. But do open up with yourself about yourself. Set yourself free!

Triggers will come up for you? That's okay. It's part of the process. Note any triggers you encountered and how you coped with them. This can help you become more aware of situations that may challenge your recovery and the strategies that work for you. Mindfulness allows you to observe these triggers without immediately reacting, providing a moment to choose a healthier response. Don't judge yourself. We cannot control our immediate thoughts, although we can change them.

Were there cravings associated with those triggers? It's okay to experience cravings, it's also part of the process. I'm 100% sober and haven't had a drop since *I Woke Up One Day & Changed My F*cking Mind* but the cravings pop up every once in a while. Not an actual physical craving but a habitual craving when it's surrounding an event, celebration or even a sunny day. The craving of the habit.

I'm observing the sensations and thoughts associated with them. I have to honour myself and allow them to arise and pass without judgment. This definitely empowers me to make conscious choices by using my mind to override the temptations.

Identify and explore the feelings you experienced during the day. Be honest and open with yourself about the highs and lows. Creating a truth, having a full understanding of oneself is liberating and exactly what I mean when I say loving yourself and returning to your source or your core.

D. Set Goals and Intentions

Set small, achievable SMART goals for yourself. Whether they are related to your recovery, personal growth, or general well-being, having goals gives you a sense of purpose and encourages you to plan a roadmap to reach those goals. Look at me! I got sober and started writing a book. A book that I have wanted to write for over a decade.

E. Celebrate Achievements

You know you are a rockstar right?

How much amazing shit have you done in your life?

Did you graduate university? Did you have children? Did you save a puppy from traffic on the road?

We tend to get so stuck in all of the nasty shit that we have done while drinking that we forget how absolutely amazing we really are.

Write all that down!

Don't believe me that you are amazing?

Let me ask you this. Who loves you?

Your mom? Dad? Kids? Spouse? Grandparents? Best Friend? Do you know why they love you? I'm willing to bet that you may not be able to answer that. If you can't, ASK THEM! Get that validation. It's important to feel validated. Have you done something to help any of those people? That's an achievement! Celebrate it!

I want you to celebrate your accomplishments, no matter how small you think they are. Recognizing and acknowledging your achievements reinforces positive behavior and boosts your confidence.

Casually running 400 meters would probably be pretty insignificant to Usain Bolt. While for us regular folk, running that same 400 metres for the first time would be a major accomplishment! Don't compare other's achievements to yours. You aren't in competition with anyone but yourself.

You don't need to justify your goals to anyone. Just set them, achieve them and celebrate them!

Then make new ones.

F. Write Letters to Yourself

Consider writing letters to yourself. You can pen encouraging notes, advice, or words of support that you can revisit during challenging times. Do you have old text messages or emails that encourage or support the type of amazing person you are? I still have all of my little folded up square notes from when I was in school from old friends/boyfriends. Find pictures of yourself with your children. The "I love you's" from your kids are enough. "I am a good mom." "I am a great dad." "I am a great parent because my kids believe in me." Simple. Your negative opinions of yourself have zero importance here. What positive things do others have to say about you? Leave the negative bullshit talk out of this.

You can consider using prompts. If you ever feel stuck, use prompts to inspire your writing. Prompts can be questions or statements that guide your thoughts. For example, "Today, I am proud of..." or "One thing I learned about myself is..." If it is hard for you to find positive things to write about, it's only because you haven't retrained your brain. You need to work on it. The past isn't going to serve you anymore. You can only use the past to learn and to grow from. We can get so stuck in who we were that we often don't believe who we are now or who we are becoming. Reprogramming and rewiring our brain takes training. Treat it like a muscle. Train your brain.

It would be pretty unrealistic to go to the gym maybe once or even 4 times and expect to have abs, now wouldn't it? So why do we put the expectation on our sobriety and our mindset that things need to change right here and right now? Stop that. Stop beating yourself up. If you just keep working at it you will get the results you want.

Remember to be kind to yourself, especially when reflecting on challenges. Hey! We've all got them. No sense in beating ourselves up. What does that do? Just makes us feel shitty. We have felt shitty long enough. It's time to reframe because we are amazing as fuck! Treat your journal as a safe space where you can express your thoughts without judgment.

Maybe you are the opposite of me and are a terrible writer but are an amazing artist. I'm a terrible artist. You can tell your story in pictures. I would be willing to bet that your pictures starting today are going to look a lot different than they will in a month or even six months from now.

I've been posting a lot of rainbows on my Instagram lately. They just keep randomly appearing in my life. I believe that I am manifesting them. Rainbows are a sign of hope, spirituality and new beginnings. Well then! *Brain Wow.* I am INCREDIBLY hopeful of my sobriety journey through the love and support that I have in my life because of others and my dedication to myself. I have definitely reconnected with my spiritual self and my soul during this whole writing process and the words flow through me. They do not come from me. I didn't make the words. I'm not telling myself what to write. Where does it come from? I am so connected to my source right now that the words are coming from Source.

If rainbows are a sign of new beginnings and I've seen 5 this week then holy moly I'm in for some major change. I remain fully open to the process and expect miracles in my life. Every day.

Go create your own rainbow!

G. Review and Reflect

It's one thing to write or draw your thoughts and/or feelings down, but to just leave them and never return to them disables you from revisiting them and seeing your growth. I mean it's not all going to be butterflies and rainbows, I get that.

When you are ready though, be sure to come back and revisit what you put down because it will surprise you immensely how far you have come. Who doesn't like to be pleasantly surprised? There in itself is something to write about (your progress).

Become your own inspiration. Periodically review your entries and reflect on your progress. This helps you track your journey, recognize patterns, and gain valuable insights into your recovery.

Make sure you stay consistent. I stopped writing for years and I felt so dead and stuck in my own mind. It's been terrible. I definitely drank more when I wasn't writing than when I was. There's another *Brain Wow* moment. By pouring my days, thoughts, ideas, achievements and goals onto paper I was "feeling" something without even recognizing it. Remember earlier I mentioned that I would drink to feel "something", "anything?"

Perhaps I could have saved myself earlier if I just stuck to what I loved and ultimately needed – writing.

I have been nose deep into this book since the middle of January (It is the middle of April now). I completely changed my patterns from drinking everyday to writing everyday. Connecting to myself has naturally connected me to something greater in the universe. I am more patient and calm with my family. I'm more understanding, I'm more outgoing. I created a new Instagram account about a month ago where I post videos several times a day. I have NEVER posted a video on social media. Ever. My oldest daughter thinks it's cringy. I'm okay with that. I have such a strong confidence and knowing that this is what I should be doing. To share my struggles and successes with my followers. I'm here to inspire, help, motivate and love others. If I can't prove that I love myself by being authentically free then how can I encourage others to do the same?

I've been so consistent in my life the past couple of months because I am so damn determined to get this book done. I feel like I owe it to my readers in a sense. Consistency has been key to reaping the benefits of journaling (creating this book). I've aimed to write regularly, even if it's just a few minutes each day. The cumulative effect of consistent journaling can be powerful. Look at all that I have accomplished just by writing a little bit each day!

I got my son back, and that's number one. There's so much more calm in the house. I'm not spending money at the casino. I've gained hours in my life because I'm not borrowing hours from tomorrow in order to ride out my hangovers. I'm sleeping better. I'm up at 4 am with a purpose. I'm stronger, I'm eating better, I'm healthier and I'm happier. I'm just a better human.

It wasn't sobriety that saved me. It was writing and truly connecting to my soul. In actuality I saved myself. That's some powerful shit right there. No one did it for me. I dug deep, I used the tools that I have set in this book and I fucking did the work.

7. Mindfulness Retreats/Workshops or Programs

Consider attending mindfulness retreats or workshops focused on recovery. These immersive experiences can deepen your understanding of mindfulness practices and provide a supportive environment for personal growth. Have you ever been on one? I haven't been on one specifically for recovery, although I have been on retreats before. The experience is almost indescribable.

To be immersed in nature with like-minded individuals who are all there for the same reason. To learn, grow, experience and gain insights into our inner self is absolutely liberating and fulfilling.

You even have the ability to enroll in structured programs like Mindfulness-Based Stress Reduction (MBSR). These evidence-based programs often incorporate mindfulness meditation and can provide comprehensive tools for stress management and relapse prevention. These can be short but intensive mini courses to really help you gain a hold on your meditation and mindful practices, encouraging you to confront and process difficult emotions. As we learn to sit with discomfort without resorting to substances, they develop resilience, which becomes a robust defense against relapse triggers.

Mindfulness nurtures emotional resilience which is a crucial aspect of maintaining sobriety from alcohol. Emotional resilience enables us to navigate challenges, manage stress, and cope with emotions in a healthy way.

Remember that cultivating mindfulness is a gradual process, and consistency is key. Start with small, manageable practices and gradually expand as you become more comfortable. Building emotional resilience is an ongoing process that evolves with time and practice. As you incorporate these strategies into your daily life, you'll likely find that your ability to cope with emotions and challenges will strengthen without resorting to alcohol. Remember that seeking support, whether from friends, family, or professionals, is a sign of strength and can significantly contribute to your emotional well-being through your journey to sobriety.

Cognitive Mindfulness

Educating myself more and more on the cognitive impacts of alcohol has really solidified my decision to put down the bottle for good. When you can learn about the cognitive aspects of addiction, understanding the cognitive processes involved in alcohol dependence can provide valuable insights into your own thoughts and behaviors.

I encourage you to practice cognitive restructuring through Cognitive Behavioral Therapy (CBT):

CBT is a therapeutic approach that helps us identify and modify unhelpful thought patterns. A trained therapist can guide you through this process. This is where we begin the cognitive restructuring by deliberately changing negative thought patterns. When you notice thoughts that may lead to relapse, challenge and reframe them with more positive and constructive alternatives.

Changing our thought patterns rather than simply sticking with routine allows us the time to consider the consequences of our choices. Being aware of the potential outcomes allows us to make decisions aligned with our sobriety goals.

Rather than going straight to the liquor store after a long day of work (like I wanted to yesterday, for a cold beer) I came home, had an amazingly delicious and healthy supper, had a bath then went to bed early without any regrets or ridiculous spending.

Changing our habits and thoughts patterns has to foster flexibility though. By being open to new ideas and perspectives, this adaptability allows us to navigate challenges more effectively and consider alternative approaches to situations. Not just with alcohol but in all aspects of our lives. We literally need to rewire our cognitive pathways so that we curb the habits and cravings and redirect our thoughts and motions towards activities that are more conducive to our goals.

Constantly consider your motivations, goals, and the progress you've made. Remind yourself daily! Many times a day. This reflective practice enhances your awareness of your journey and the cognitive processes at play.

Your goals fucking matter! If you don't take SMART actions to achieve those goals, they are just wishes. We did that when we were children. Now we take action to make shit happen!

Go Make Shit Happen!

CHAPTER 23
Self-Reflection

This section can be a bit tricky to get through. We're going to really get the gears going here to come to a deep understanding of how the fuck did we get here? Why the fuck did we start drinking?

Self-reflection becomes a compass for navigating the intricacies of the past, unearthing the root causes of alcohol abuse. It can help prompt us to explore underlying traumas, unresolved issues, and ingrained beliefs that may have contributed to our relationship with substances.

Tapping into the root causes of any substance abuse disorder is a crucial step in understanding the underlying factors that contribute to addictive behaviors. Exploring these root causes can provide insights into the origins of our relationship with alcohol, enabling us to address the core issues and support our recoveries.

I've compiled some strategies to help you identify and understand some of the root causes of why you drink.

Self-Reflection

Dedicate time to self-reflection. This goes hand in hand with the mindful meditation practices. Consider your life experiences, relationships, and significant events. Reflect on how these factors may have influenced your relationship with alcohol. Don't forget to journal these reflections. It's important to remember and reflect on your past but not to STAY there!

Alcohol can no longer be the protagonist in your life's story. It is important to recognize how your relationship with alcohol is evolving. You CAN heal and move on with your life. Don't sit in that space anymore. YOU are now the protagonist in your own life!

Therapy and counseling in the past couple of years has been instrumental in my recovery process. Seeing my therapist during the thick of it and continuing to see her as I am now sober. It's always nice to have a third party to help me discuss and reflect on everything that has gone on and is going on in my life.

Professional support provides a safe and structured space to explore our past, like our childhood experiences where we can examine family dynamics. Early life events and family environments can significantly impact our relationship with substances. We can learn to identify any traumatic experiences, family dysfunction, or patterns of behavior that may have contributed to our alcohol use.

We may have had trauma, whether physical, emotional, or psychological. This can unknowingly be a root cause of addiction because we used alcohol or other substances as coping mechanisms. Specialized therapeutic approaches can help address trauma-related issues. Going through a complete history of your past can leave clues on how you got here.

Seeking therapy can help you to recognize the coping mechanisms you developed throughout your life or mechanisms you used to deal with your family history of addiction if any. There may be genetic and environmental factors that contribute to addictive tendencies. Understanding your family's history with substance abuse can provide additional context.

Understanding how alcohol became a coping mechanism for stress, anxiety, or unresolved emotions is best discovered with help. If you have been doing this without help. How is that working for you? I encourage you to seek therapy. I am a huge advocate of therapy. I believe that everyone can benefit. I actually get excited about my sessions now.

23. Self-Reflection

Analyzing your behavioral patterns, especially those related to stress, emotions, relationships and identifying any recurring themes or triggers that lead to alcohol use. You may not even know what these are. We can get so stuck in our habits and our patterns that we may not even recognize behaviors or patterns that lead us to drink.

Having help to unravel them is instrumental to recovery.

Perhaps you may have some co-occurring disorders such as anxiety, bipolar or depression. In my personal opinion I would seek help from a psychiatrist, psychologist or therapist who is aware of your alcohol use and who is familiar with the effects of long-term alcohol use. A professional who can work with you in your recovery HAS to have knowledge in the field of recovery. By understanding the intricate connections between mental health and substance use, trained and licensed professionals can implement strategies that foster dual recovery, promoting overall well-being.

The correlation between mental health issues and alcohol abuse is well-established, and the relationship is complex and multidirectional. Individuals with mental health disorders may turn to alcohol as a means of self-medicating, while excessive alcohol use can contribute to the development or exacerbation of mental health issues. This is key information here!

I said how much I love my therapist and how she has been a key player in my sobriety as a sounding board to get the ugly shit out. She is a Certified Trauma Professional and a Registered Therapeutic Counsellor.

Never once did she put me on a treatment plan or try to get me off of alcohol. She acted as a "Talk Therapist" for me. Which is totally fine and I am so grateful for her. A psychiatrist is a medical doctor who has access to more resources to help facilitate a treatment plan for recovery and who understands the physical and mental effects of long-term alcohol use and how alcohol can be a cornerstone for the physical/mental challenges of anxiety, bipolar and depression.

As I had mentioned before, alcohol was 100% responsible for my depression and anxiety. I didn't learn this through therapy. I learned it on my own by really doing the ugly work which ultimately turned out to be beautiful.

In conjunction with working with a psychiatrist or therapist, beginning to engage with support groups such as Alcoholics Anonymous (AA) or SMART Recovery may be a good fit for you as well. This is the same acronym that we used before in achieving goals but in this context it refers to Self-Management and Recovery Training. AA takes a more spiritual approach to recovery while SMART Recovery takes a more scientific approach to recovery. Trying one or both may be beneficial so that you find what works for you. They are both programs with high success rates for helping others with their sobriety.

I encourage you to educate yourself in the process. I'm a student of life for life. I just love to learn and I continually have my nose in a book or course.

Don't shy away from reading literature on addiction, psychology, and recovery. Knowledge about the science of addiction and psychological processes can empower you to understand the root causes on a deeper level and what you can do for yourself and others. My ultimate goal here is to pass the torch. I want you to get so right in your head and in your sobriety that you become a beacon for others to turn to. I want my journey to have a snowball effect and to trickly down the line.

One Person At A Time.
You
Are
Next
It's your turn!

23. Self-Reflection

Consider Life Transitions

Do you ever find yourself going for the bottle or engaging in self-destructive behaviour because of major life experiences? Remember when I talked about being pregnant with my baby LunDhyn and how he definitely saved my life after my dad died? I know without a doubt I would have completely spiralled out of control immediately following my dad's death. In hindsight I think I didn't truly grieve the loss of my dad to its full capacity because I was so concerned with the pregnancy. I tried to remain as calm as possible. My obstetrician did give me medication to deal with the loss of my dad. I didn't take it. I wanted my dad, not drugs.

Yes, I cried of course, but I didn't get deep with myself and actually grieve. I suppressed so much. I guess subliminally, I tried to set myself up to deal with it later. I had a new baby coming into the world. I didn't have "time" to process my dads passing.

I definitely lost my shit after my youngest son was born and spiralled so far down that I contemplated taking my own life.

So we know that death can definitely be a trigger. What about other losses like a divorce, a break up or even a career change? As far back as I can remember. I don't recall receiving a manual or training on how to deal with loss, even though we can begin to experience it at such a young age and just be expected to know how to deal with it.

Brain Wow moment here – why in the fuck are we not talking about loss at a younger age? Like what to expect, what to avoid, what we are going to feel. I believe that more education is definitely needed here in order to give people tools and resources to turn to and use for when these life changing events happen.

Say you have been at your job for twenty five years. Same thing day in and day out. You then get laid off. Now what?

You are just supposed to go through life like nothing happened? This is a HUGE event that needs to be handled with love, compassion, therapy and a plan. It should be treated as a death. It certainly acts as one. Major events in our lives produce major emotions like stress, anxiety, boredom, loneliness, or sadness that may trigger the desire to drink. Emotional triggers are often key contributors to alcohol use. When you can really get a grip on your triggers which leads to an understanding of your emotions when in turn leads to a better connection and understanding of yourself.

John and our life together was definitely a trigger for me. He wasn't going to break the pattern of going to the liquor store first. He wasn't going to break the pattern of asking me if I wanted more booze when he would see the bottle getting low. If he wasn't then who was?

Me, myself and I. That's who!!

I didn't need him to quit in order for me to quit. It actually worked the other way. I made the decision that I was done and he followed suit. I'm proud of him.

That's some powerful shit right there.

I have the ability in me to change not only my life – but 5 other lives as well...

Reflect on your relationships and how they impact your alcohol use. Consider whether specific people, conflicts, or dynamics contribute to drinking. Understanding relationship patterns can reveal important triggers. Be your own boss of your life. Don't wait for others to change.

> "We but mirror the world. All the tendencies present in the outer world are to be found in the world of our body. If we could change ourselves, the tendencies in the world would also change. As a man changes his own nature, so does the attitude of the world change towards him. This is the divine mystery supreme. A wonderful thing it is and the source of our happiness. We need not wait to see what others do."
>
> – Mahatma Gandhi

23. Self-Reflection

It's important to protect your emotional state by setting boundaries with yourself and others. We tend to do things we will later regret when we are vulnerable.

Yes, it is true that we need our people within our sobriety but remember that not everyone is on the same journey as you so please consider social situations that prompt drinking. This could include gatherings with certain friends, celebrations, or events where alcohol is readily available. Social triggers can play a significant role in patterns of alcohol use. Take a funeral for example. Yes it is important for you to attend if you feel called to do so, what is not important is for you to stay at the reception and drink. You are allowed to leave. Did you hear that?

You.

Are.

ALLOWED.

To.

Leave.

No explanation needed. Taking control of the things you can means that you are training your mind to accept you for who you truly are and to trust yourself. If you have ANY sticky feelings about being in a place where there is alcohol, you need to leave.

That sticky or uneasy feeling is your sign to go.

It's okay to….

Go.

CHAPTER 24

Overcoming Obstacles

Relapse sucks.

There's no two ways around it. This time for me is the last time I am "getting sober."

I have quit drinking in my life more times than I can count.

This time is for good.

How did I get to this point that seems to be so hard for so many?

Mindfulness and self-reflection has been paramount in my recovery. I make it a priority with no questions asked that my mental state comes first. Before my work, my kids or my husband. I don't just practice this when I'm triggered or stressed, I practice it all day.

I'm glued into my motivational audio books. I'm writing this book, which is the ultimate journaling. I make it a priority to remain as peaceful and understanding as possible with those who are around me. I stretch. I focus on my breathing techniques. I'm creating new patterns and routines in my home. I'm focused on my life being smooth and controlling what I can and letting go of what I can not. I am constantly practicing gratitude either in my head, heart or out loud. I make it a priority to give thanks every single day for my home. The brand new home that I was able to acquire for my family through the thick of my habitual addiction.

That doesn't mean that my life is now perfect. I am absolutely triggered some days when I'm encountered with stressful situations or have a long day at work, or if I'm at a restaurant and the server asks me if I want a drink. Of course I want a fucking drink. I do now, however, have an absolute knowledge that drinking in moderation doesn't work for me. I can NEVER have just one. Having "just one" is a subliminal promise my mind has made to my body, so I have rewired my mind to promise my body to just never have "just one." It took work and it will continue to take work. I'm committed to my new job.

Just because someone offers you alcohol you CAN say "NO." "Why not?" should be removed from our vocabularies. Why do we deceive ourselves? We know exactly why we should not! Stick with that truth!

Emotional and Physical Responses. It's impossible (at least from my past experience) not to feel a strong sense of guilt and shame after a relapse. Understand that these emotions are natural but also recognize that they can hinder your progress. Be compassionate with yourself. Write it down, talk about it, why? How do you justify your relapse? Is your answer completely ridiculous? Probably, right? Unless it's physical where the withdrawal is overwhelming and alcohol is the only way to feel "normal" and to make the physical symptoms go away you need to quit again… Never quit quitting.

Please seek medical intervention if you are in the early stages of sobriety and have a physical dependency on alcohol which is severely disabling your ability to stay sober. In-patient rehab may be a good fit for you.

There is absolutely nothing wrong with professional help. It doesn't make you look weak, you don't look stupid. I promise! It makes you look strong and in control of your life. You are making the decision that alcohol doesn't get that front seat in your life anymore. You are more powerful than the alcohol.

It's okay to admit you can't do it alone. That would be a pretty huge endeavor – that no one should be expected to take on by themselves. You know you can't do it alone. You may be a professional drinker and may not be a professional in sobriety (yet) so seek out those professionals. As with anything we want to learn to do, we seek out support/teachers/professionals.

Use your relapse as an opportunity for learning. Understand what went wrong, what you can do differently in the future, and how you can strengthen your recovery plan.

Did you set an unrealistic goal? Was it SMART (sustainable, measurable, attainable, realistic, time sensitive)? Did you go from 24 beers a day, going to the pub every day after work to nothing? That is not a SMART goal approach at all. I know what you are thinking... "All or nothing." Sometimes for some people "all or SOMEthing may be more manageable." I did relapse many times over the years, until I didn't because *I Woke Up One Day & Changed My F*cking Mind*. There will come a time when you relapse for the last time because your life is more important than the alcohol in your life. We HAVE to stop giving it so much power.

Going from that example to complete sobriety is doing a 180 in your life. Literally everything has to change.

The people involved, the location, the time spent, the food eaten, the routine of going to the pub everyday, coming home and drinking more until you black out and do it all again tomorrow.

We talked about rewiring the brain. The brain likes routine, consistency and reliability. When you have been doing the same thing for so long it can feel impossible to get out of it, even if it's toxic for us. Like a nasty relationship.

It takes time to form new habits. Give yourself the time.

Let's take that example and make it SMART.

1. Instead of going to the pub after work just go home! Well stop at the liquor store first for a 12 pack. Seriously... break the first physical routine. If you don't start here you will make it harder than it has to be.

We are already winning because of the amount of money you will have saved by not going to the bar and buying less.

2. What do you do when you drink at the bar? Talk? Great! Call someone. Pick up the phone. Have a beer in your hand. That's fine. Enjoying the conversation? Can you actually hear the person on the other line because you aren't screaming over other people or the music?

Bartenders watch you like a hawk when you're drinking. They have the next one lined up before you have your last one finished. We equate this to "excellent service." How loose do your pockets get for that "excellent service" by the end of the night? That's all it is. We tip more and order food when we are drinking. The booze you consume only benefits the house staff, not you. On top of that! The price of alcohol at a bar is absolutely astronomical!

3. Cook for yourself. Can't cook? That's fine. Learn! There are billions of recipes online. I have Googled a couple of times a few ingredients that I had in my house and I was surprised with the ideas that google came up with for me to make, with what I had.

We all love to eat. There's something so satisfying about cooking for yourself or your family a delicious meal. Remember we are rewiring and learning new coping mechanisms and skills. Make food for the soul.

I could keep going on how to do this but I think you get the point. Changing our patterns and social circles is an absolute priority in order to get a grip of this thing.

You HAVE to stay committed to this! Reaffirm your commitment to sobriety. Understand that recovery is a journey with its ups and downs. Use your experiences as motivation to recommit to your goals. I wholeheartedly use my past experiences with alcohol as motivation not to drink again.

It's okay to adapt and modify your plan or your SMART goals. Be flexible and willing to adapt as needed. If certain aspects of your plan are not effectively preventing relapse, consider modifying them in collaboration with your support network.

24. Overcoming Obstacles

Recovery is a process, and setbacks do not erase the progress you've made. Reaffirm this for yourself! "Setbacks do NOT erase the progress that I have made."

Use a relapse as an opportunity for growth, learning, and refining your approach to sobriety.

Handling societal pressures while trying to stay sober from alcohol can be challenging, but it's crucial for your recovery. Celebrate your sobriety milestones openly. Communicate your achievements to friends and family, emphasizing the positive aspects of your journey. This can foster a supportive atmosphere.

Remember Your Why!

Why is sobriety important for you?

I don't want to hear "because of my kids." As we know I've got four, but I didn't get sober for my kids. I got sober for me. My sobriety and the benefits from it are a byproduct for my children. I got sober because I felt like I was dying. I got sober because there is so much I want to do. I got sober so I didn't gamble anymore. I got sober so that I can lose weight. I got sober so I can be of service to others. I got sober so I can be healthy. I got sober so I can be truly authentically me. I got sober so I can be a more present mother. I got sober so that I can get to know who I am.

I keep my reasons for staying sober at the forefront of my mind. I remind myself of the positive changes and benefits I've experienced since choosing a sober lifestyle. I wouldn't change one day of sobriety for another drunken night at the casino. Ever!

I'm continuing to build a life that is in line and congruent with my goals and values.

I got sober for me!

I know you can do this! You are LIVING and breathing proof that if you couldn't do this you wouldn't be here today. So how about that!

Now you go do you, boo!

CHAPTER 25
Have The Best Day Ever!

Wow! I can't believe that I'm here and that I got to the last chapter. Thank you for getting here with me. Thank you for being with me as I move through my sobriety.

As I got to this page this morning a sense of calm and excitement flowed through me. I FUCKING DID IT!

Not only did I not have one drop of alcohol since *I Woke Up One Day & Changed My F*cking Mind…* I wrote a fucking book!!!

Something that I had been thinking about for 10 years, I accomplished in three months (91 days to be exact).

I am living proof that dreams and wishes stay as such unless you take action.

That's what I did! I took action and look at where I am now.

There is absolutely no way I could write any book, let alone one on sobriety if I was still drinking. I had a one-track mind and it was to get to the bottom of the bottle.

I am now commanding and demanding the time in my life that I want to focus on things that fulfill my heart and my soul. Physically I've done a 180. My anxiety is gone, mentally I am as sharp as a whip, emotionally I am free – my depression is gone, spiritually I have found peace. When the mind can start to see and think straight the soul reemerges.

From the beginning, I had all of my chapters laid out with bullet points for the content I wanted to expand on. That's it. Out of the goodness of the universe, the words just came through me to fill in the blanks. They definitely didn't come from me. It was effortless. I didn't question myself once as I put these words on paper. I now have a complete understanding that I have done the right thing and that sharing my story, my wisdom and my heart with the world is an act of service which will touch many people for generations to come.

I hope that I have made an impact in your life albeit small or large. Alcohol is all around us, one way or another. It is never going to be far from our periphery. That is a fact.

What is also a fact is that you have the power and the strength inside of you to conquer alcohol and to live your very best life. Don't place blame. Remember that you with alcohol is not the real you! It chemically changes who you are.

It is imperative that you don't go through this alone. Find your community. If you can't find one, make one! I have learned that sober people are just so incredibly inspiring, enlightening, loving and kind.

Getting sober is like flicking a switch. The byproducts of quitting is awakening, rising up to all that life has to offer, with grace, ease, determination, strength and love.

I started writing this book in order to document the process of my sobriety, then I began to realize the social norm of alcohol use and abuse, especially amongst my fellow '90s girls and how "wine o'clock" became its own digit.

If I was struggling so much with this physical, mental and emotional push and pull then others must have been as well. And what about the next generation? Are they going to be as fucked up as mine? Not if I have anything to do with it.

If I would have had some of the tools available to me when I was in high school and in my 20s I would have known better and done better.

The tools are here and available for you now! It's not too late. I'm sorry it took me so long.

It is my goal and my ultimate desire that this book of transformation has been and will continue to be a message of overcoming what seems to be insurmountable obstacles. A

25. Have The Best Day Ever!

message of hope, love, dedication to yourself and your family. Not only did I quit drinking but I changed my life by using all of the tools in this book.

In my experience It is 95% mind work and 5% physical work. Your body will do whatever the mind tells it to.

Take these tools and apply them, take action and you will begin to see the life you were leading unfold into a clean slate with the past drifting away as it no longer serves you.

I know that you can get through this similarly to how I did!

I have faith that you will grow and become all that this amazing universe has set out for you to be.

You matter! You are important! You are worthy! You are loved!

Learn these lessons, practice these lessons, own these lessons then the rest is history and you are free!

It's time to close that book, and now mine because you need to go have a glass of water, put on your shoes, get outside and start connecting to your soul! Find beauty every step of the way.

As I say, "Goodbye", I hope that you too are able to say …

"I Woke Up One Day & Changed My Fucking Mind"!

I love you and hope you have the BEST day ever!

Love,

Challaine

A Letter To My Beautiful Children

My letter to you:

NiKylo, PaLoma, JorDhyn and LunDhyn aka Big Guy, Boba, Button and Bubzee/Lunny.

You four humans are my world. I love you more than anything.

NiK and Loma, I was twenty-three and twenty-six when I had you. Your father and I were the BEST of friends. He saved me from a toxic relationship that probably would have killed me. I loved him very much, and he loved me back.

We were still kids when we had you. Trying to figure out the ropes of our own lives separately and together, then trying to figure it out again with babies.

I don't want you to think for one second that us separating had anything to do with you. I promise – it didn't.

We had gotten to a point in our relationship where I felt I couldn't mother him anymore. I was making more money, I had the license, the rent was in my name, I had the credit cards, I had the motivation and drive to grow and learn. We weren't equals in the relationship, not by a long shot. I didn't mind carrying more of the load as I was able and happy to at the time but it began to get frustrating when I was the only one in our relationship who had the umph to get up and go. I couldn't keep carrying more of the load, forever.

I took on so much more that maybe there was some unintentional, subconscious resentment there for that. I wanted such great things for us, but because of his past and lack of willingness to learn and expand his horizons we were limited to options together as a family. "As a family" got awkward. It felt forced. That's when I knew.

I had to ask him to leave. It broke his heart and it broke mine. I lost my best friend, my protector, my guy, but I outgrew him and had to think about what was best for me and you two. I know without a doubt I did the right thing.

Your father is one of the greatest men I have ever known, and he still is to this day (even though we don't communicate as much anymore. I'll assume his core is just more of what it was). I see his love for your two. It makes me so happy that your relationship with him is strong. You all need each other.

He loves hard, he's brutally honest (a little forgetful), a big teddy bear, tremendously tough, generous, kind, loving, emotional and funny as hell. He's one of the VERY few men who could make me belly laugh. I am grateful for our 7 years together. I am grateful that I have you two because of him.

Being a new mom to you two, working on my career as a Personal Trainer, expanding my education, trying to get my own finances together, it was a lot!

I will always hold a place in my heart for your dad. He has always meant well with you and loves you so much it makes him cry. He just didn't have it in him to be present and parent the way he needed to or be the partner I needed him to be. He WANTED to, though, but just didn't have the tools. We had the discussion several times that it would be best for him to stay away until he "got his shit together" or at least, "got a vehicle"…

Unfortunately, so much time had gone by until he was able to do that. Now, as you know he is happy in his relationship with his partner and has great bonus kids AND a relationship with you guys now. Everyone gets along. You share your lives with each other. You are happy where you are at and as you get older I know it will continue to grow. Keep working on it! It's important.

I mean what more could I ask for in an ex? To be honest, your dad is pretty much the perfect ex for me. He has trusted me to mother you, to raise you, provide for you, make the decisions for you. For that I am so grateful.

I hope that you never hold resentment towards him for not being around. I hope that you don't have resentment towards me for asking him to leave.

I promise you my loves, that it was one of the best decisions for me to make, for me, for you and ultimately him.

For this, I give thanks.

They always say, "Make sure you are ready before you have kids." Are you ever "ready"? Well, at the time of writing this, I've had four kids and I promise you, you are NEVER ready. That definitely does not mean for one instant that you were never wanted, or second guessed. It just means that every child is different and there is absolutely no way you could ever know how to handle or what to do with that child because every single one is unique. I have learned that a baby just communicates with its mother what they need. Without words. Mums have this innate intuition that guides us along until children are able to communicate more effectively what they need or want.

So without you here, how could I be ready for you?

I remember my life without you but I could NEVER imagine my life without you.

Since I was a little girl I knew I was going to be a mom. NiK, I had your name picked out in junior high school, if not elementary. You were named after Nick Carter – the Backstreet Boy. No it's not lame, he was literally one of the most famous guys on the planet to MILLIONS for more reasons than one. You, my son, are a jaw dropper.

NiKylo – You are so incredibly talented in your athleticism. I feel it in my soul that you are going to make it to the big leagues. Your hard work, dedication and love for the game is incomparable to anything I've ever seen. Since you were first on skates playing Timbits hockey and you scooted around with your "running skate" to now, is incredible. Your coaches have always been your fans. They admire you and are rooting for you to go all the way. We all are. This year playing juniors is a huge milestone for which you should be so proud. Going to Latvia at this age is insane!

I am beyond proud of you. I'm thrilled to see you excel at what you love. You do it with your ego aside, with love for the game and with respect for others. I couldn't be more proud of the baby you were, the child you grew into, the young man you have become. You are incredibly smart, funny, loving, sensitive, so helpful and strong.

You are my firstborn and NOTHING will ever change that. Does that make you my favorite? No, lol – it doesn't – it does mean though that I had you to myself for three years. There is something special in that. We had so much "you and me" time. I loved you and wanted you before I was pregnant with you. I miss the little you, A LOT. Tears are filling my eyes as I write this. I miss our time together, our hugs, cuddling in bed, your little voice. One thing that I will always have is the memories of us when you were little.

Witnessing the young man that you are today, I've done an amazing job. The point is for you to grow up and start your own life. Nothing will make that easier for me but to watch you grow and just be the amazing human you are makes me so undeniably proud.

I am so sorry that you had to be witness to my years of drinking. I was feeling that I was losing you. I know you were too. Even though I know you were mad at me, thank you for always loving me. I'm proud of you for standing up to me and deciding not to put up with my bullshit anymore. I need you, for always.

You are perfect for me and I love you.

<u>PaLoma</u> – My first daughter.

Oh, my beautiful girl, who lives in a smile. You are the apple of my eye, you are my little bestie who likes to push my buttons but all in all you are absolutely incredible and I adore you.

I admire you – your fearlessness, your confidence, your grit, your attitude and your strength. When you set your mind to something you go out and get it done. Except cleaning the bathroom lol.

You are a brilliant artist. Keep working on your art and expanding your mind through your creativity. You have genius in you. I hope the whole world gets to see.

You are so kind, gentle, incredibly patient (I could learn a bit of this from you). You are an amazing friend to others, your connection with animals is adorable.

You are the most EXTRAORDINARY big sister to the littles. They love you so much! Thank you from the bottom of my heart for being there for them when I couldn't; either mentally, physically, or because I was on the road for work. I'm sorry that you saw me drunk on more than one occasion. At first I know you didn't really "get it" but as you got older and started to understand what "getting drunk" was and started comparing me to other moms who drank, it didn't take you long to catch on what being drunk was and seeing me with alcohol would eventually lead to me being drunk. I'm sorry.

I just love you, my Boba.

I hope you have children one day. You will be a better mother than most mothers I know, and most certainly me. I hope I have set you up with some of my strengths to carry you forward in this world and that you have seen my weaknesses and have learned from them… My weaknesses have become my strengths. I'm confident yours will too.

Please know that I'm doing better now because I know better and have done a crazy amount of work to get where I am. Please continue to come to me with what's going on in your life. I love you and want to be here for you. Always!

I know you will continue to handle life with class, tenacity, a firm stance which is backed by resilience and love for the world around you.

If you don't have kids, I will be sad, not disappointed. I will respect your decision and have solace in knowing that whatever you do in your life you will go above and beyond and will be one of a kind.

I named you after my best friend in high school. She is bright, creative, kind, loving, and loves her cats lol. She is spiritually connected and a queen in my eyes. I hope as you get older maybe you two could connect. I'm so excited for your future and what you are going to bring to this world. It will only be for the greater good!

Keep spinning my beautiful girl

Never stop dancing and sing loud even when you don't know the words

You are perfect for me and I love you

TO BOTH OF YOU

I am so sorry for not having my head screwed on tight for all these years. I've experienced a few significant traumas and losses in my young life, and it appears that I have subconsciously turned to alcohol to just make me feel good rather than going through the motions while seeing the beauty and joy in the day to day.

You are old enough now to know when mum has been drinking, you have both called me out on it. Unfortunately, you will have these memories for the rest of your lives and for that I'm incredibly sorry. I pray that you don't carry with you in your life "my mother was an alcoholic" and have this as your "childhood trauma." I want the world for you two and I hope that the good that I have done for you will outweigh the excess of booze in my life and yours.

I hope that you see the struggle with alcohol abuse that I had over the years and steer clear away from it in excess. I hope you have learned some things from this book about your mum. I am human. I am always trying to figure it out and get it right but I'm certainly not perfect.

You guys will make mistakes, BIG ones. Use them as opportunities for self-reflection, for growth, for change so you can be better and to learn from them.

That's what I did.

Don't beat yourselves up for your mistakes. It's okay. I promise. Learn and move on.

I love you two so much. Thank you so much for being you.

Continue to be each other's best friends – NiiiiiiK (I know you heard that while reading it) lol. She's your little sister and she needs you – even when you're rich and famous and all the girls are after you. Loma comes first. ALWAYS make time for her.

There may be a time again when you are all that you have. Your bond is special.

I love you, guys, so much, and remember to…. Have The Best Day Ever!

Love,

Mommy

JorDhyn and LunDhyn

You two render me speechless.

I was 35 when I had you JorDhyn and Lunny I was 37 when I had you.

NaNa was 36 when she had me, and your amazing Gramps (rest his beautiful soul) was 49 when I was born. I was always the one with the "old parents." Having a mother with a disability rendered me embarrassed a lot of the time, shamed, I felt like I didn't fit in. My mum never really hung out with my friends parents – they didn't have much in common with the age difference and NaNa having MS…Multiple Sclerosis.

Having a mother with a disability was really hard for me but it was the only life I knew. As an only child it was up to me to do what she couldn't, which was LOTS. I grew up faster than I had to because I was put (unintentionally) in a position at a very young age where I had to parent the parent. I remember times when my mum would have an exacerbation from the MS and I was sent away to stay with a family friend because she couldn't cook for me, do the laundry, or drive me to my activities. She was sometimes hooked up to IV Prednisone and just had to ride it out.

I tried to be a "good girl" because high stress can cause an exacerbation and I didn't want it to be my fault that she would get sick. I tried but it didn't always work out that way – I was …

Just.

A.

Kid.

There were times when I was sent away to the children's cottage in Calgary where children would go when their parents "needed a break." My mum really thought I was out of control, but I had so much on my plate between being a kid, school, my activities, the chores, taking care of her… and, and, and. We never talk about childhood stress but it's a real thing and it definitely played out in my behaviour at home.

Even though I am older having you two, I don't want you to be ashamed of having me as your mum, I don't want you two to feel sad that I'm older and that you are going to miss out on the "good" years with me.

You two earth angels came into my life at the perfect time. I think I need you more than you need me.

You have given me a renewed purpose. NiK and Loma – don't take that the wrong way lol. You two are part of my purpose every single day but as you get older, more independant and become free, you need me less and less. It's my harsh reality.

JorDhyn – Dad and I met May 12th 2017 and were engaged October 26th 2017. I had left a previous relationship of five years to be with your dad. The breakup was sad and messy but my heart led me to him, and we moved in together, Jan 2018. Dad moved into my condo, which became our condo. After living in the condo for a year we moved to a house down the street where the bigs would have their own rooms upstairs with us…. Then in 2020 I got pregnant with you, NiK moved to the basement and there was a little bedroom at the end of the hall ready for your arrival.

BEFORE YOU WERE HERE

Dad and I would sit outside almost every night (drinking usually) and go on and on, back and forth about having another child.

I was hesitant because it meant another c-section, it meant starting all over again. My babies were out of diapers… Oh!!!! The diapers.

We both wanted more kids. Daddy unofficially adopted your brother and sister but never had his own biological kids. I was the person to give him that.

I always wanted a big family because I never had that. It was always just me and NaNa. Mum and Dad are both only children.

So in 2020 after a couple of years, I just made an executive decision and went to the doctor, got my IUD taken out and I was pregnant the same week.

OMG! Thank you thank you thank you! I was absolutely ecstatic

I was so excited. We called you Jem when you were on the inside as we knew you were going to be JorDhyn Emerson McNally. You were our little Jem.

I do need to mention my beautiful Button, that you are a twin. We lost your brother or sister early on in the pregnancy. I'm not a twin (obviously) and I don't know too many but maybe just keep that piece of information close to you as you navigate this world.

JorDhyn – Your brilliance is outstanding. You are wise beyond your years (at only 2). You are absolutely beautiful and have such a big and loving heart. You are really shaping up to be an amazing big sister to your little brother and it makes me so proud. I often wonder what you are going to do with those incredible brains of yours. A scientist? A doctor? A business owner? A Lady Boss? I think you already own that title and wear that crown proudly.

Every day you amaze me beyond words and I'm so happy that you chose me to be your mummy. Gramps is so proud of you. He met you when you were teeny tiny and loves you so much.

Thank you for being you.

You are perfect for me and I love you.

LunDhyn

My baby boy. Oh, my beautiful baby boy. My momma's boy. How could I be so blessed to have 2?

You have only been on the outside for a short while. At the writing of this book you are 1 year and almost 4 months young. You started walking this past Christmas while "That's Christmas to me" was playing in the background in our big new beautiful Christmas house. I burst into tears. It is a moment I will never forget.

Having you has brought me so much joy. You are so gentle and loving, quiet, inquisitive, silly, incredibly handsome and just a joy to have around. I hate leaving you and being on the road. I miss you so much.

Before I got pregnant with you, I had a miscarriage. They are always blessings in disguise. As heartbreaking as it was at the time I knew we were going to try again. I was terrified during my pregnancy with you. I didn't want to lose another one. I wanted you so bad.

You never got to meet your Gramps. He passed away May 19, 2022 a few months before you were born in October. He was so happy and excited to be a gramps for the 4th time. I have pictures of him holding my belly – which was you.

After you were born it felt like a piece of my dad was reincarnated into your soul. You possess so many of his amazing qualities already. He was an amazing man, my best friend and my hero. He loves you.

As I watch you navigate the world with laughter, love and the young hunger to shoot the puck, I feel so blessed to be able to witness your little gears turning to learn the world around you.

Thank you for choosing me to be your mummy.

You are perfect for me and I love you.

<u>To Both Of You</u>

You two are so lucky to have each other and to be so close in age. You will be each other's best friends for life. JorDhyn, as his big sister it's your responsibility to have his back, but Lunny as the man, you make sure you protect her with all your heart.

I feel like having you two has given me the chance to start over with this whole parenting thing. Not that I completely screwed it up with NiK and Loma. I only knew what I knew but now I know better.

I promise to be more present mentally and physically. I promise to not lead the life I was living before.

I promise to not let myself go so that you feel shame, extra responsibility or embarrassed by me. One thing I cannot control is my age but one thing I can control is how I treat my body and move forward in this world.

I look forward to the many years to come where I get to see you two thrive and grow into the amazing humans I know you are destined to be. Kind, compassionate, caring, loving, inspirational and just incredible.

<u>TO ALL OF YOU</u>

No matter where this life leads me, no matter what mistakes I make (I'm bound to make more) and no matter the distance, know in your hearts that I am always with you. NiK, I'm always cheering you on as you play, PaLoma I'm always a phone call away for ANYTHING. JorDhyn – I'm excited to see where our journey leads us together and Lunny – don't ever stop being a momma's boy, no matter the distance…

Now go on you four ….

Get.
Go.
And.
Have the BEST day ever!

Love,

*Mummy, Mom, Mother,
Mama, Dada (lol), Bruh, Pookie*

Acknowledgements

To everyone that I have hurt over the years. I am so incredibly sorry. I ask for your forgiveness. I ask for forgiveness from my friends, family, clients, co-workers, even the cop I was so mean to the night I got arrested.

I want to offer an extended thank you and ask for forgiveness from my in-laws. They flew all the way across the country to be here for our family and to help us raise their grandchildren. I'm so sorry for all of the chaos. You didn't deserve that! Amidst it all you were always there for me (us) and loved me unconditionally. Maybe there were a few conditions lol but you loved me regardless. Thank you! And thank you for being the best Gran and Grandpa to my bigs. They need you just as much as the littles. They are all incredibly lucky to have you in their lives. So am I.

Thank you a million times over for everything. I love you!

To all of my teachers I thank you. Wayne Dyer, may you continue to rest in peace. You have been my saviour for many events in my life where I was drowning. Without your wisdom, love and support through the messages in your books, where I am now, would definitely not be possible. We all need a village. Thank you for being a part of mine.

When I saw you walk out on stage a few years ago it felt like God walked out. I now know it wasn't a feeling. It was a knowing. I'm so glad I got to shake your hand and pass you the letter I wrote to you.

I love you!

Mel Robbins…

Thank you for being my North Star! You have been such a support in my ear as I keep you glued in while I'm working. I have gained so much confidence and wisdom listening to you and your guests.

"In case no one told you today...
I love you and I believe in you!"

To you! Yes, you reading this book! I freaking love you, I'm so proud of you and I can't wait to see and hear where this life takes you. I know you are going to rise from the ashes and shine bright. I want to thank you for taking this journey with me and helping me get through the toughest of the tough. Knowing that in order to be strong for me I had to be strong for you. I have created my own community to help me. Remember I said earlier, if you didn't have friends or a support system, to go find one! Just like I did here. I found you and you found me. We did not meet by accident!

I hope this book serves as a beacon and tool of hope, transformation, wisdom and strength for my generation and those to come. Come back to this often. Use the tools inside these pages. I am a living and soulfully happy truth that the words within these pages aren't just text, they are medicine for your life.

It is my commitment to stand with you and beside you as you go through your journey of sobriety. I have an absolute knowing that you have greatness to give to this world because you ARE greatness! We can only give what we possess. I am grateful for you!

Johnny Boi!

John, you are such an amazing husband to me and father to our kids. The way you have unofficially adopted the bigs, you have done seamlessly. I feel that maybe because you were adopted you just have a bigger heart and are just more loving and accepting. You NEVER say, "Your kids." All four are yours/ours.

Even though we have had a terribly tumultuous past, we are here now.

ACKNOWLEDGEMENTS

We have literally been to the depths of hell together. I can confidently say that we are at peace, in love and amazing parents together with undeniable teamwork and partnership like nothing I have ever seen or experienced.

My ex was the love of my life at the time and took up a lot of space in the beginning of our relationship. I'm sorry for that.

My soulmate is you John, without a doubt. I know that because I hate you many days but wouldn't choose not to have you any day. I don't want to do this life without you.

I'm looking forward to this next chapter. Look how far we have come in 91 days!

I love you, Moose!

Challaine…

I'm so fucking proud of you for finally kicking the bottle to the curb.

I'm proud of you for doing the work
I'm proud of you for your determination
I'm proud of you for reaching your goals
I'm proud of you for the mother you are
I'm proud of you for your strength
I'm proud of you for asking for help
I'm proud of you for being a support to others
I'm proud of you for all of your accomplishments
I'm proud of you for honouring your word
I'm proud of you for your honesty
I'm proud of you for your transparency
I'm proud of you for your resilience
I'm so fucking proud of you for writing your book
I love you…
Now go on you…
You've got more goals to crush!
But before you go make sure you take this with you…
"Have The Best Day Ever"!

Love,
Challaine

www.ingramcontent.com/pod-product-compliance
Lightning Source LLC
Chambersburg PA
CBHW052134070526
44585CB00017B/1819